Genetic Engineering: Properties, Structures and Functions of DNA

ABOUT THE AUTHORS

Maninder Singh is Post Graduate in Biotechnology from Multanimal Modi College, Modinagar and submitted Ph.D. in Biotechnology from C.M.J University Shillong, Assam. Presently he is working as a lecturer in Biotechnology Department at Dr. K.N. Modi Institute of Pharmaceutical Education and Research, Modinagar District, Ghaziabad, Uttar Pradesh. He has attended various seminars and conference presented International papers.

Alis John has obtained M.S. and Ph.D. in 1995. His professional career began at London, where he and his colleagues worked on DNA sequencer and Synthesizer and the Protein synthesizer, In addition to having published more than 380 per reviewed articles, he has coauthored textbooks in biochemistry, immunology, molecular biology and genetics, as well as popular book on the human genome projects, The Code of Codes.

ABOUT THE BOOK

Genetic engineering has allowed scientists to change an organism's looks or function by adding, deleting, or rearranging genes. Genetic engineering is based on an understanding of the molecular aspects of genetic processes occurring in nature. The techniques of gene manipulation enable us to transcend conventional biological boundaries to create completely novel gene combinations and even new genes. Deoxyribonucleic acid, or DNA, is a biological macromolecule that carries hereditary information in many organisms. DNA is necessary for the production of proteins, the regulation, metabolism, and reproduction of the cell. Large compressed DNA molecules with associated proteins, called chromatin, are mostly present inside the nucleus. Some cytoplasmic organelles like the mitochondria also contain DNA molecules. This book provides a concise introduction to all the key topics of genetic engineering and background information to the reader intent to understand this fascinating subject. This book presents the principles of gene manipulation and its associated techniques in sufficient details and also covers biological replication of DNA, protein synthesis and its regulation, nucleic acid, ribonucleic acid, restriction endonuclease, tools and manipulation, regulation, application and vaccines etc.

Genetic Engineering
Properties, Structures and Functions of DNA

Maninder Singh
Alis John

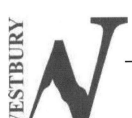

WESTBURY PUBLISHING LTD.

ENGLAND (UNITED KINGDOM)

Genetic Engineering: Properties, Structures and Functions of DNA
Edited by Maninder Singh & Alis John
ISBN: 978-1-913229-45-0 (Hardback)

© 2020 Westbury Publishing Ltd.

Published by Westbury Publishing Ltd.
Address: 6-7, St. John Street, Mansfield,
Nottinghamshire, England, NG18 1QH
United Kingdom
Email: - info@westburypublishing.com
Website: - www.westburypublishing.com

British Library Cataloguing in Publication Data:
A catalogue record for this book is available from the British Library.

For more information regarding Westbury Publishing Ltd and its products, please visit the publisher's website- www.westburypublishing.com

Preface

Genetic engineering has allowed scientists to change an organism's looks or function by adding, deleting, or rearranging genes.

The term 'genetic engineering' stands for human alteration of the genetic code of an organism, so that its biosynthetic properties are changed. The major applications are for the industrial production of desired peptides or proteins, or to alter the biological capabilites of the organism. These techniques have been used to develop crops with agronomically useful changes, such as pest resistance and ripening properties that allow for shipment. Surprising results have been obtained by silencing genes in experimental organisms, as well as the production of animal models of human disease by deriving strains of animals with mutated human genes.

Genetic engineering, also called genetic modification or genetic manipulation, is the direct manipulation of an organism's genes using biotechnology. It is a set of technologies used to change the genetic makeup of cells, including the transfer of genes within and across species boundaries to produce improved or novel organisms. New DNA is obtained by either isolating and copying the genetic material of interest using recombinant DNA methods or by artificially synthesising the DNA. A construct is usually created and used to insert this DNA into the host organism. The first recombinant DNA molecule was made by Paul Berg in 1972 by combining DNA from the monkey virus SV40 with the lambda virus. As well as inserting genes, the process can be used to remove, or "knock out", genes. The new DNA can be inserted randomly, or targeted to a specific part of the genome.

Genetic engineering has been applied in numerous fields including research, medicine, industrial biotechnology and agriculture. In research GMOs are used to study gene function and expression through loss of function, gain of function, tracking and expression experiments. By knocking out genes responsible for certain conditions it is possible to create animal model organisms of human diseases. As well as producing hormones, vaccines and other drugs genetic engineering has the potential to cure genetic diseases through gene therapy. The same techniques that are used to produce drugs can also have industrial applications such as producing enzymes for laundry detergent, cheeses and other products.

DNA is usually a double-stranded polymer of nucleotides, although single-stranded DNA is also known. Nucleotides in DNA are molecules made of deoxyribose sugar, a phosphate and a nitrogenous base. The nitrogenous bases in DNA are of four types – adenine, guanine, thymine and cytosine. The phosphate and the deoxyribose sugars form a backbone-like structure, with the nitrogenous bases extending out like rungs of a ladder. Each sugar molecule is linked through its third and fifth carbon atoms to one phosphate molecule each.

DNA was isolated and discovered chemically before its functions became clear. DNA and its related molecule, ribonucleic acid (RNA), were initially identified simply as acidic molecules that were present in the nucleus. When Mendel's experiments on genetics were rediscovered, it became clear that heredity was probably transmitted through discrete particles, and that there was a biochemical basis for inheritance. A series of experiments demonstrated that among the four types of macromolecules within the cell (carbohydrates, lipids, proteins and nucleic acids), the only chemicals that were consistently transmitted from one generation to the next were nucleic acids.

This is a reference book. All the matter is just compiled and edited in nature, taken from the various sources which are in public domain.

This book provides a concise introduction to all the key topics of genetic engineering and background information to the reader intent to understand this fascinating subject.

—*Editor*

Contents

(viii)

1

Introduction

TECHNOLOGY OF GENETIC ENGINEERING

Genetic engineering is a radical new technology, one that breaks down fundamental genetic barriers — not only between species, but between humans, animals, and plants. By combining the genes of dissimilar and unrelated species, permanently altering their genetic codes, novel organisms are created that will pass the genetic changes onto their offspring through heredity.

Scientists are now snipping, inserting, recombining, rearranging, editing, and programming genetic material. Animal genes and even human genes are being inserted into plants or animals creating unimagined transgenic life forms. For the first time in history, human beings are becoming the architects of life. Bio-engineers will be creating tens of thousands of novel organisms over the next few years. The prospect is frightening.

Genetic engineering poses unprecedented ethical and social concerns, as well as serious challenges to the environment, human health, animal welfare, and the future of agriculture. The following is just a sampling of concerns:

Genetically engineered organisms that escape or are released from the laboratory could wreak environmental havoc. Genetically engineered "biological pollutants" have the potential to be even more destructive than chemical pollutants. Because they are alive, genetically engineered products are inherently more unpredictable than chemical products — they can reproduce, migrate, and mutate. Once released, it will be virtually impossible to recall genetically engineered organisms back to the laboratory. A report published by 100 top American scientists warned that the release of gene-spliced organisms "...could lead to irreversible, devastating damage to the ecology."

Gene-splicing will likely result in unanticipated outcomes and dangerous surprises. Biotechnology is an imprecise science and scientists will never be able to ensure a 100 per cent success rate. Serious accidents are bound to occur. Researchers conducting experiments at Michigan State University recently found that genetically altering plants to resist viruses can cause the viruses to mutate into new, more virulent forms, or forms that can attack other plant species. Some other scary scenarios: foreign genes from genetically engineered plants could be carried by pollen, insects, wind, or rain, and flow into other crops, as well as wild and weedy relatives. Disaster would follow if genetically engineered crop traits, such as insect and virus resistance, found their way into weeds, for instance.

Genetically altered plants could produce toxins and other substances that might harm birds and other animals. Genetic engineering of plants and animals will almost certainly endanger species and reduce biological diversity. By virtue of their "superior" genes, some genetically engineered plants and animals will inevitably run amok, overpowering wild species in the same way that introduced exotic species, such as kudzu vine and Dutch elm disease which have created problems in North America. What will happen to wild species, for example, when scientists release into the environment carp, salmon, and trout that are twice as large, and eat twice as much food, as their wild counterparts? Another danger lies in the creation of new kinds of crops and domesticated animals. Once researchers develop what is considered to be the "perfect tomato" or "perfect chicken" these will be the ones reproduced in large numbers; "less desirable" species would fall by the wayside. The "perfect" animals and plants could then be cloned (reproduced as exact genetic copies), reducing even further the pool of available genes on the planet.

Genetically engineering plants to be herbicide-tolerant will lead to increased use of chemicals in agriculture and further contamination of the environment. Biotech companies love to say that genetic engineering will end the use of dangerous chemicals in agriculture. But the leaders in biotechnology are the giant chemical companies like Monsanto, Du Pont, and Rhone-Ponlenc; they aren't interested in losing profits from the sale of chemicals. These companies are genetically engineering plants to be resistant to herbicides that they manufacture so they can sell more herbicides to farmers who, in turn, can apply more poisonous herbicides to crops to kill weeds. In fact, crops genetically engineered to be herbicide-tolerant account for nearly half of the applications for field testing submitted to the U.S. Department of Agriculture (USDA) since 1988. Even genetically engineering crops to produce their own pesticides presents dangerous problems. Pests will eventually evolve that are resistant, then stronger chemicals will be needed to get rid of the pests. And what will happen when the pesticide gene spreads to weeds and other unwanted plants? The genetic engineering of crops and food-producing animals can produce toxic and allergic reactions in humans. Someone allergic to peanuts or shellfish, for example, would have no way of knowing if a tomato or other food had been altered with proteins from these substances, and could have a fatal reaction by eating such genetically altered foods. In addition, genetic engineers can take proteins from bacteria they find in the soil, the ocean — anywhere — and incorporate them into human food. Such substances have never been in the food supply before, so their toxic or allergenic characteristics are unknown.

Genetically engineered products do not have a good track record for human safety. In 1989 and 1990, a genetically engineered brand of L-tryptophan, a common dietary supplement, killed more than 30 Americans and permanently disabled or afflicted more than 5,000 others with a potentially fatal and painful blood disorder, eosinophilia myalgia syndrome, before it was recalled by the FDA. The manufacturer, Showa Denko K.K., Japan's third largest chemical company, had used genetically engineered bacteria to produce the over-the-counter supplement. It is believed that the bacteria somehow became contaminated during the recombinant DNA process. There were no labels on the product to identify the product as having been genetically engineered.

The patenting of genetically engineered foods, and widespread biotech food production, will eliminate farming as it has been practiced since the beginning of humankind's appearance on the planet. If the trend is not stopped, the patenting of transgenic plants and food-producing animals will soon lead to tenant farming in which farmers will lease their plants and animals from biotech conglomerates and pay royalties on seeds and offspring. Eventually, within the next few decades, agriculture will move off the soil and into biosynthetic industrial factories controlled by chemical and biotech companies. Never again will people know the joy of eating naturally produced, fresh foods. Hundreds of millions of farmers and other workers worldwide will lose their livelihoods. The hope of creating a human, sustainable agricultural system will be destroyed.

The genetic engineering and patenting of animals reduces living beings to the status of manufactured products and will result in much suffering. In January 1994, then-USDA Secretary Mike Espy announced that USDA scientists had completed genome "road maps" for cattle and pigs, a precursor to ever more experimentation on live animals. In addition to the cruelty inherent in such experimentation (the mistakes are born with painful deformities, crippled, blind, and so on), these "manufactured" creatures have no greater value to their "creators" than mechanical inventions. Animals genetically engineered for use in laboratories, such as the infamous "Harvard mouse" which contains a human cancer-causing gene that will be passed down to all succeeding generations, were created to suffer.

A purely reductionist science, biotechnology reduces all life to bits of information (genetic code) that can be arranged and rearranged at whim. Stripped of their integrity and sacred qualities, animals who are merely objects to their "inventors" will be treated as such. Currently, more than 200 genetically engineered "freak" animals are awaiting patent approval from the federal government. No one is regulating genetically engineered organisms adequately or properly testing them for safety. In 1986, Reagan-era policymakers stitched together a patchwork of pre-existing and only marginally appropriate statutes to ease the way for new biotechnology products. But these laws were created years ago to deal with chemicals — not the unpredictable living products of genetic engineering. To date, no suitable government apparatus has been set up to deal with this radical new class of potentially overwhelming environmental and health threats.

The FDA's policy on genetically altered foods illustrates the problem. In May 1992, then Vice President Dan Quayle, and head of the Competitiveness Council, announced the U.S. Food and Drug Administration's newly developed policy on biotech foods: genetically engineered foods will not be treated differently from naturally produced foods; they will not be safety tested; they will not carry labels stating that they have been genetically engineered, nor will the government keep track of foods that have been genetically engineered. As a result, neither the government nor consumers will know which whole or processed foods have been genetically engineered.

Vegetarians and followers of religious dietary restrictions face the prospect of unwittingly eating vegetables and fruits that contain genetic material from animals — including humans. And health risks will be discovered only by trial and error — by consumers. USDA oversight is no better. This agency has the conflicting task of both promoting and regulating agriculture, including genetically engineered plants and animals used for food. Indeed, the USDA is a primary sponsor of biotech research on plants and animals.

By patenting the genes they discover and the living organisms they create, a small corporate elite will soon own and control the genetic heritage of the plant. Scientists who "discover" genes and ways of manipulating them can patent — and thus own — not only genetic engineering techniques, but the very genes themselves. Chemical, pharmaceutical, and biotech companies such as DuPont, Upjohn, Bayer, Dow, Monsanto, Cib-Geigy, and Rhone-Poulenc, are urgently trying to identify and patent plant, animal, and human genes in order to complete their take-over of agriculture, animal husbandry, and food processing. These are some of the same companies that once promised a carefree life through pesticides and plastics. Would you trust them with the blueprints of life?

Genetic screening will likely lead to a loss of privacy and new levels of discrimination. Already, people are being denied health insurance on the basis of "faulty" genes. Will employers require genetic screening of their employees and deny them work on the basis of the results? Will the government have access to our personal genetic profiles? One can easily imagine new levels of discrimination being directed against those whose genetic profiles reveal them to be, for example, less intelligent or predisposed to developing certain illnesses. Genetic engineering is already being used to "improve" the human race, a practice called eugenics. Genetic screening already allows us to identify and abort fetuses who carry genes for certain hereditary disorders. But within the next decade, scientists will likely have a complete map of the human genome to work with. Will we abort fetuses on the basis of non-life-threatening impairments such as myopia, because someone is predisposed towards homosexuality, or for purely cosmetic reasons? Researchers at the University of Pennsylvania have applied for a patent to genetically alter sperm cells in animals so traits passed down from one generation to the next can be changed; the application suggests that this can be done in humans too.

Moving from animal eugenics to human eugenics is one small step. Everyone wants the best for their children; but where do we stop? Inadvertently, we could soon make the efforts of the Nazis to create a "superior" race seem bumbling and inefficient.

The U.S. military is building an arsenal of genetically engineered biological weapons. Although the creation of biological weapons for offensive purposes has been outlawed by international treaty, the U.S. continues to develop such weapons for defensive purposes. However, genetically engineered biological agents are identical whether they are used for offensive or defensive purposes. Areas of investigation for such weapons include: bacteria that can resist all antibiotics; extra-hardy, more virulent bacteria and viruses that live longer and kill faster; and new organisms that can defeat vaccines or natural human or plant resistances. Also being studied are the development of pathogens that can disrupt human hormonal balance enough to cause death, and the transformation of innocuous bacteria (such as are found in human intestines) into killers. Some experts believe that genetically engineered pathogens that can target specific racial groups are being developed as well.

DEVELOPMENT OF GENETICS

The significance of Mendel's laws was not recognised by his contemporaries but became evident 35 years later, just after the turn of the twentieth century. At this time other important events marked the progress of genetics: Sir Archibald Garrod, a physician, made important contributions to the chemistry of diseases especially porphyria, cystinuria and alkaptonuria, noting their recurrence among sibs in the same family and the effect of consanguineous marriage. He introduced the term "inborn errors of metabolism" and the concept of "one gene, one enzyme" and thus opened the way to biochemical genetics, which became one of the most important aspects in the development of genetics.

Theodor Boveri and Walter's. Sutton in 1903 independently proposed the chromosome theory of inheritance, stating that the chromosomes carried the "hereditary factors" proposed by Mendel and that their behaviour during cell division provided an explanation for their segregation during meiosis. In the twentieth century the fruit fly, Drosophila was the organism most extensively used in the study of genetics. It was extremely useful because it was easily bred in the laboratory, reproduced very rapidly (about 20 times in one year) and produced thousands of offspring that could be analysed. Besides, it had only four chromosome pairs that were exceptionally large in the salivary glands and showed a pattern of transverse bands on which individual genes could be localised.

THOMAS HUNT MORGAN is one of the most famous of the hundreds of scientists who worked on Drosophila. He described sex-linked characteristics that were manifest in the male flies. He is best known for proposing methods for estimating distances between genes located on the same chromosome through the phenomenon of recombination. The unit of gene distance, the centimorgan, is named after him. Morgans work opened up the important field of gene mapping.

Advances in human genetics did not parallel the great advances in the genetics of Drosophila since the beginning of the twentieth century.

This was mainly due to:

• The inability to perform breeding experiments in man;

- The very long generation time
- The small size and relatively large number of human chromosomes, which made their microscopic examination very difficult.

However, several hundreds of human genes were known to exist through the visible characteristics they produced. In the 1950s two great advances completed the phase of growth of classical genetics and paved the way for a new era of genetics.

The molecular structure of DNA, which explained how the molecule could replicate itself and how the same molecule could represent an almost infinite variety of different genes. From then the gene could be visualised as a structural entity and was no longer an invisible hereditary particle that could be identified only by its effects on the characteristics of an organism. The discovery of the molecular structure of DNA thus paved the way for the study of the gene itself and the direct analysis of DNA in the new era of molecular genetics that was to follow. TIJO and LEVAN devised a technique for the study of human chromosomes and established that the human chromosome number was 46. Earlier techniques were suitable for organisms that had few chromosomes but not for human chromosomes, which were small and numerous. This was immediately followed by the discovery of chromosomal abnormalities and marked the beginning of human cytogenetics. It was one of the most important advances that brought human and medical genetics into prominence.

The New Genetics

A new era of genetics began in the 1970s with the development of three new techniques, which together enabled the direct analysis and manipulation of genes. At this stage studies on DNA were performed mainly on bacteria as they had a very short generation time and very simple DNA. Most of the new discoveries arose from the study of bacterial genetics. Hamilton Smith discovered that bacteria produced "restriction endonucleases", enzymes that had the ability to cut open the DNA molecule at specific sites.

ED Southern at Edinburgh University developed a technique by which specific genes could be isolated from the whole complement or genome of DNA. The process was called Southern blotting.

Stanley Cohen at Stanford University developed the use of plasmids, which are naturally occurring circular loops of DNA capable of entering bacterial cells, as vectors for carrying foreign DNA into bacterial cells.

These three techniques of cutting, isolating and inserting genes form the basis of recombinant DNA technology, popularly called genetic engineering.

They also formed the basis of modern genetic technology. We are now on the threshold of a new era that promises the treatment of genetic diseases.

PRESENCE OF A GENETIC EFFECT

The presence of a genetic effect was originally established for activity through selective breeding of animals showing high activity scores, low activity scores, or both on a standardized measuring technique. One of the earliest attempts to establish the hereditary basis of activity using this method was a selection study by Rundquist, in which he selected rats for high and low activity following testing in an activity wheel.

His results were disappointing initially, because of an error in the method of selection he employed: the mating of high active and low active offspring from nonselected parents. That is, rats showing high activity scores were selected not only from parents that also had high activity scores, but from those yielding low activity scores as well, with the reverse holding true for rats with low activity scores. As a result, there was no differentiation between groups from generations F_1 to F_4. When this error was corrected, differentiation into high and low active groups did occur and laid the foundation for further research in this area.

Hall performed selection experiments in the early 1930s to establish the genetic basis of emotionality in rats using as phenotypes the Behaviour of the rats in an open field. Although he was not concerned with activity per se, his selection procedures and his use of the open field test have served as the prototype for many of the modem studies on this problem.

In the 1950s, it became possible to use another method for determining hereditary basis for activity and for any other phenotype. This method involves finding differences in activity between strains of genetically controlled animals, usually highly inbred strains of mice and rats, but also established breeds of dogs and inbred strains of various species of *Drosophila*. Thompson tested five strains of inbred mice on two activity measures, the open field and the Y maze. His results showed marked differences in the activity levels of the five strains, and the two C_{57} strains showed much higher activity levels in both open field test and the Y maze than did the BALB/c mice.

In mouse studies, McClearn has shown that there is a clear relationship between locomotor activity and the percentage of $C_{57}BL/Crgl$ genes present (from backcrosses with A/Jax mice). Thompson illustrated that there is considerable variability between strains in exploratory activity, with $C_{57}BR/a$, $C_{57}BL/6$, and $C_{57}BL/10$ having the highest mean score (for activity) and A, AK/

e, and BALB/c strains having the lowest. These orderings were fairly invariant with another testing apparatus (enclosed arena versus Y maze). There are differences in the ordering of mice on exploratory activity with different environmental conditions. For example, he found that in bright white light, A/Crgl mice showed less exploratory activity than in dim red light. In the C_{57}BL/Crgl mice, activity increased in white light and decreased in dim red light. Although he found no change in the ordering of the strains, McClearn did find a significant interaction between strain and illumination.

Of particular historic and current interest are the MR and MNR rats originated by Broadhurst. Using a procedure essentially similar to that used by Hall more than two decades earlier for selection for emotionality, Broadhurst made several important improvements; the open field was more uniformly and brightly lighted and initial responses of the subjects were weighted more heavily, giving less emphasis to the possible adaptation of the rats to a familiar environment. MR and MNR rats clearly differ on open field defecation scores, an index of emotionality, and are often regarded as "benchmark" strains for this category of Behaviour. However, on several *activity* measures, these strains do not differ greatly. Selection studies illustrating genetic differences in activity have also been carried out in species other than rats and mice.

The comparison of the normal Behaviour of different established breeds of dogs provides an excellent example; for "everyday" differences in activity levels, one need only compare a bassett hound and a fox terrier. Dogs have also been used as subjects in more systematic genetic studies, with different breeds treated analogously to inbred strains of rodents.

A prime example of this sort of research is the 19 year study conducted by Scott and Fuller that dealt with, among other things, the emotional Behaviour of several breeds of dogs, together with their hybrids and backcrosses. Clear genetic differences were found in the five breeds on a variety of reactivity tests, including open field Behaviour. Some work on activity and its implications has also been done with the fruit fly. In one study flies were selected for mating speed. Activity differences for these two selected strains (fast mating speed and slow mating speed) were measured by counting the number of squares a fly entered in an open field arena over a given period of time. It was found that slow mating lines exhibited more open field activity than did fast mating lines.

In contrast, Ewing, in selecting for spontaneous activity, found that the less active lines displayed *more* sexual Behaviour than did the more active lines. Although these results appear to contradict Manning's findings, the discrepancy appears to have been due to an "apparatus effect," as he used an apparatus other than the open field used by Manning. When Ewing replicated his study using the type of open field apparatus used by Manning, no significant differences between the selected lines were found.

Besides being alterable by apparatus effects and other environmental changes, activity is readily changed, often differentially for different genotypes, by internal events, especially pharmacological agents. A thorough review of drug effects on activity, and the genetic factors involved, has recently been prepared by Broadhurst. The studies we have cited are typical of many others to be found in the literature, in that many of the findings are contradictory with one another, with varying differences among genotypes (whether inbred strains or selected lines) depending on procedural details, types of apparatus, and so on. Therefore, generalizations on activity levels of specific genetically controlled animals should be treated cautiously.

An excellent example illustrating this point can be found in an article by Lassalle and Le Pape. They demonstrated that the environmental conditions associated with testing of two inbred mouse strains ($C_{57}BL/6$ and BALB/c) can reverse the general finding we referred to earlier that C_{57}s are more active than BALB/cs. Under seminatural and breeding cage conditions, the BALB/cs showed a higher level of activity than did the C_{57}s, and in the seminatural condition, the BALB/cs were more active in the dark).

In an issue related to the genetic determination of activity, several studies have attempted to determine heritabilities and degrees of genetic determination. However, as these findings are limited to the specific genetic population measured within a specific type of apparatus and a specific set of environmental conditions, these data are of rather limited use in the generalizable information they provide for an understanding of the genetic basis of activity.

POLYGENIC MODELS

There are various avenues of research that have suggested that a polygenic model can best account for activity. One form of evidence for this type of genetic determination can be found in score distributions; typically, a continuous, unimodal distribution of scores has been found for most types of activity measurement when genetically heterogeneous animals were tested.

Tryon suggests a polygenic model on the basis of this form of evidence alone. An excellent example of a more thorough analysis supporting a polygenic model can be found in the series of studies reported by DeFries and Hegmann. They tested large numbers of two inbred strains of mice ($C_{57}BL/6J$ and BALB/cJ), as well as their reciprocal F_1 and F_2 hybrids and backcrosses.

The mice were tested for 3 minutes on each of 2 successive days in an automated, white Plexiglas open field, 90 cm². The means and variances of the transformed scores. The degree of increase in variance from the F_1 to the F_2 generation is inversely related to the number of loci affecting a trait. The variance between the F_1 and F_2 generations is very slight, especially when compared with the difference in variances between the parental strains and the F_1 generation. (One can discount the variance"differences between the reciprocal F_2 s as a maternal effect, especially as it diminishes in later generations.) DeFries and Hegmann conclude that activity is controlled by genes at several loci, suggesting *at least* 3.2 loci from an earlier analysis by Hegmann.

A "mineral occurrence" is a concentration of a mineral (usually, but not necessarily, considered in terms of some commodity, such as copper, barite or gold) that is considered valuable by someone somewhere, or that is of scientific or technical interest. In rare instances (such as titanium in a rutile bearing black sand), the commodity might not even be concentrated above its average crustal abundance.

A "mineral deposit" is a mineral occurrence of sufficient size and grade that it might, under the most favourable of circumstances, be considered to have economic potential. An "ore deposit" is a mineral deposit that has been tested and is known to be of sufficient size, grade, and accessibility to be producible to yield a profit. (In these days of controlled economies and integrated industries, the "profit" decision may be based on considerations that extend far beyond the mine itself, in some instances relating to the overall health of a national economy.)

On one hand, the field observations usually begin with "mineral occurrences" (or with clues to their existence) and progress with further study to "mineral deposits" and only rarely to "ore deposits," but we must present information that helps us deal with all classes of "mineral occurrences," not just "ore deposits." On the other hand, in terms of accessible information our sample is strongly biased toward "ore deposits," for it is only in them that sufficient exposure is available to develop a real knowledge of the overall character of the mineralization process. Some mineral occurrences are, therefore, unrecognized mineral deposits, while others are simply mineralized localities where ore forming processes were so weak or incomplete that a deposit was not formed. Thus we summarize the state of knowledge regarding ore deposit models, and we call them "mineral deposit models" with the hope that what we have learned about large and high grade metal concentrations will help us sort out all mineral occurrences to identify their true character and, we hope, to recognize which have potential to constitute ore deposits.

The attributes or properties of a mineral occurrence are, of course, those features exhibited by the occurrence. When applied to a model, these terms refer to those features possessed by the class of deposits represented by the model. It is useful to consider attributes on at least two scales: the first deals with local features that may be observed directly in the field (mineralogy, zonal patterns, local chemical haloes, and so on); the second is those features concerning the regional geologic setting and which must be interpreted from the local studies or may be inferred from global tectonic considerations (for instance, that the rock sequence under study represents a deep water, back arc rift environment, or that the area is underlain by anomalously radioactive high silica rhyolite and granite). Two of the most prominent attributes, the commodities/geochemical patterns and the mineralogy, are cross indexed to model types.

To the greatest extent possible, models were constructed so as to be independent of site specific attributes and therefore contain only those features which are transferable from one deposit to another. This goal is difficult to attain, because we do not always know which features are site specific.

The term "model" in an earth science context elicits a wide variety of mental images, ranging from the physical duplication of the form of a subject, as in a scale model of the workings of a mine, to a unifying concept that explains or describes a complex phenomenon.

In this context we shall apply only the latter usage. Therefore, let us propose a working definition of "model" in the context of mineral deposits, the overriding purpose being to communicate information that helps mankind find and evaluate mineral deposits. A mineral deposit model is the systematically arranged information describing the essential attributes (properties) of a class of mineral deposits. The model may be empirical (descriptive), in which instance the various attributes are recognized as essential even though their relationships are unknown; or it may be theoretical (genetic), in which instance the attributes are interrelated through some fundamental concept.

One factor favouring the genetic model over the simply descriptive is the sheer volume of descriptive information needed to represent the many features of complex deposits. If all such information were to be included, the number of models would escalate until it approached the total number of individual deposits considered.

Thus we should no longer have models, but simply descriptions of individual deposits. Therefore, the compilers must use whatever sophisticated or rudimentary genetic concepts are at their disposal to distinguish the critical from the incidental attributes.

It is commonly necessary to carry some possibly superficial attributes in order not to preclude some permissible but not necessarily favoured, multiple working concepts.

One of the commonly accepted attributes of the model for the carbonate hosted lead zinc deposits of the Mississippi Valley type is the presence of secondary dolomite. But do we know that this is essential? Suppose a deposit were found in limestone; would we reject its assignment to the Mississippi Valley class? Or could it be correct that the critical property is permeability and that the formation of dolomite either:

- Enhances permeability (and thereby makes the ground more favourable),
- Reflects pre-existing permeability that is exploited by both the dolomite and the ore?

Model Names

Each model has been assigned a name that is derived either from the special characteristics of the classes or from a type locality. The latter strategy was employed to avoid excessively long descriptive names. The use of type names derived from specific deposits does produce confusion in some readers, however, who may feel, for example, that a deposit that does not look "exactly" like Comstock cannot be represented by a "Comstock epithermal vein" model.

This confusion may be minimized by realizing that most models are blends of attributes from a large number of deposits and that the names are only conveniences, not constrictions. The contributors to this report and the literature in general are not without disagreements regarding nomenclature (as well as genetic aspects and some facets of the groupings made here), but provision for alternative names is made in the model format under the heading of approximate synonyms.

Descriptive Models

Because every mineral deposit, like every fingerprint, is different from every other in some finite way, models have to progress beyond the purely descriptive in order to represent more than single deposits.

Deposits sharing a relatively wide variety and large number of attributes come to be characterized as a "type," and a model representing that type can evolve. Generally accepted genetic interpretations play a significant role in establishing model classes. Here we shall emphasize the more descriptive aspects of the deposits because our goal is to provide a basis for interpreting geologic observations rather than to provide interpretations in search of examples. The attributes listed are intended to be guides for resource assessment and for exploration, both in the planning stage and in the interpretation of findings.

The descriptive models have two parts. The first, the "Geological Environment," describes the environments in which the deposits are found; the second gives the identifying characteristics of the deposits.

The headings "Rock Types" and "Textures" cover the favourable host rocks of deposits as well as source rocks believed to be responsible for hydrothermal fluids which may have introduced epigenetic deposits. "Age" refers to the age of the event responsible for the formation of the deposit. "Tectonic Setting" is concerned with major features or provinces (perhaps those that might be portrayed only at 1:1,000,000 or smaller scale), not ore control by structures that are local and often site specific. "Associated Deposits" are listed as deposits whose presence might indicate suitable conditions for additional deposits of the type portrayed by the model.

The second part of the model, the "Deposit Description," provides the identifying characteristics of the deposits themselves, particularly emphasizing aspects by which the deposits might be recognized through their geochemical and geophysical anomalies.

In most cases the descriptions also contain data useful in project planning for mineral assessment or exploration; this aspect is especially important where limited financial and manpower resources must be allocated to the more significant tasks.

GENE LINKAGE

A chromosome has many thousands of genes; there are an estimated 100,000 genes in the human genome. Inheritance involves the transfer of chromosomes from parent to offspring through meiosis and sexual reproduction. It is common for a large number of genes to be inherited together if they are located on the same chromosome. Genes that are inherited together are said to form a linkage group. The concept of transfer of a linkage group is gene linkage. Gene linkage can show how close two or more genes are to one another on a chromosome. The closer the genes are to each other, the higher the probability that they will be inherited together. Crossing over occurs during meiosis, but genes that are close to each other tend to remain together during crossing over.

Sex Linkage

Among the 23 pairs of chromosomes in human cells, one pair is the sex chromosomes. (The remaining 22 pairs of chromosomes are referred to as autosomes.) The sex chromosomes determine the sex of humans. There are two types of sex chromosomes: the X chromosome and the Y chromosome. Females have two X chromosomes; males have one X and one Y chromosome. Typically, the female chromosome pattern is designated XX, while the male chromosome pattern is XY. Thus, the genotype of the human male would be 44 XY, while the genotype of the human female would be 44 XX (where 44 represents the autosomes).

In humans, the Y chromosome is much shorter than the X chromosome. Because of this shortened size, a number of sex-linked conditions occur. When a gene occurs on an X chromosome, the other gene of the pair probably occurs on the other X chromosome. Therefore, a female usually has two genes for a characteristic. In contrast, when a gene occurs on an X chromosome in a male, there is usually no other gene present on the short Y chromosome. Therefore, in the male, whatever gene is present on the X chromosome will be expressed.

DNA Defined

During the 1950s, a tremendous explosion of biological research occurred, and the methods of gene expression were elucidated. The knowledge generated during this period helped explain how genes function, and it gave rise to the science of molecular genetics. This science is based on the activity of deoxyribonucleic acid (DNA) and how this activity brings about the production of proteins in the cell. Genetic material is packaged into DNA molecules. DNA molecules relay the inherited information to messenger RNA (mRNA) which, in turn, codes for proteins. This chain of command is represented as:

The flow of information from DNA to protein is known as the *Central Dogma* of molecular biology. In 1953, two biochemists, James D. Watson and Francis H.C. Crick, proposed a model for the structure of DNA. (In 1962, they shared a Nobel Prize for their work.) The publication of the structure of DNA opened a new realm of molecular genetics. Its structure provided valuable insight into how genes operate and how DNA can reproduce itself during mitosis, thereby passing on hereditary characteristics. Not only did the new research uncover many of the principles of protein synthesis, but it also gave rise to the science of biotechnology and genetic engineering.

DNA Structure

As proposed by Watson and Crick, deoxyribonucleic acid (DNA) consists of two long nucleotide chains. The two nucleotide chains twist around one another to form a double helix, a shape resembling a spiral staircase. Weak chemical bonds between the chains hold the two chains of nucleotides to one another.

A nucleotide in the DNA chain consists of three parts: a nitrogenous base, a phosphate group, and a molecule of deoxyribose. The nitrogenous bases of each nucleotide chain are of two major types: purines and pyrimidines. Purine bases have two fused rings of carbon and nitrogen atoms, while pyrimidines have only one ring. The two purine bases in DNA are adenine (A) and guanine (G). The pyrimidine bases in DNA are cytosine (C) and thymine (T). Purines and pyrimidine bases are found in both strands of the double helix.

The phosphate group of DNA is derived from a molecule of phosphoric acid. The phosphate group connects the deoxyribose molecules to one another in the nucleotide chain. Deoxyribose is a five-carbon carbohydrate.

The purine and pyrimidine bases are attached to the deoxyribose molecules, and the purine and pyrimidine bases are opposite one another on the two nucleotide chains. Adenine is always opposite thymine and binds to thymine. Guanine is always opposite cytosine and binds to cytosine. Adenine and thymine are said to be complementary, as are guanine and cytosine This is known as the principle of complementary base pairing.

DNA Replication

Before a cell enters the process of mitosis, its DNA replicates itself. Equal copies of the DNA pass into the daughter cells at the end of mitosis. In human cells, this means that 46 chromosomes (or molecules of DNA) replicate to form 92 chromosomes.

The process of DNA replication begins when specialised enzymes pull apart, or "unzip," the DNA double helix. As the two strands separate, the purine and pyrimidine bases on each strand are exposed.

The exposed bases then attract their complementary bases. Deoxyribose molecules and phosphate groups are present in the nucleus. The enzyme DNA polymerase joins all the nucleotide components to one another, forming a long strand of nucleotides.

Thus, the old strand of DNA directs the synthesis of a new strand of DNA through complementary base pairing. The old strand then unites with the new strand to reform a double helix. This process is called *semiconservative replication* because one of the old strands is conserved in the new DNA double helix.

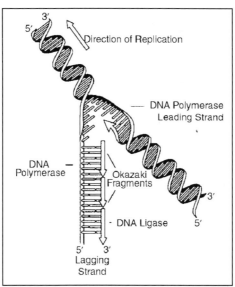

*Fig. **DNA replication. The double helix opens and a complementary strand of DNA is synthesised along each strand.***

DNA polymerase joins nucleotides in a 52-32 direction on the leading strand, shown in Figure. However, DNA polymerase does not elongate a DNA strand in a 32-52 direction. Therefore, the 32-52 strand, called the lagging strand, is synthesised in short segments in a 52-32 direction. These short segments placed on the lagging strand are Okazaki fragments and are ultimately joined together by the enzyme DNA ligase to form a new DNA strand.

DNA replication occurs during the S phase of the cell cycle. After replication has taken place, the chromosomal material shortens and thickens. The chromatids appear in the prophase of the next mitosis. The process then continues, and eventually two daughter cells form, each with the identical amount and kind of DNA as the parent cell. The process of DNA replication thus ensures that the molecular material passes to the offspring cells in equal amounts and types.

Some Basic Definitions

The genetic material is contained within the nucleus of all cells. It consists of extremely fine thread-like structures composed of DNA and associated proteins. Within it is stored the genetic information, a whole library of genes which constitute the genome.

These thread-like structures become visible as chromosomes during cell division as they gradually coil up and become thick and prominent.

For the purpose of analysis the chromosomes can be arranged as a karyotype. They are classified in order of decreasing size and according to their pattern of bands.

Chromosomes occur in pairs. There are 23 pairs of chromosomes: 22 pairs of autosomes and one pair of sex chromosomes.

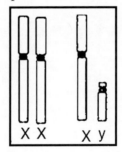

Fig. The sex Chromosomes are XX in Females and XY in Males.

The Y chromosome is much smaller than the X chromosome. It carries the genes responsible for the male sexual characteristics. The X chromosome carries genes that are not related to sex and are equally important in both males and females.

The genetic material is made of DNA. The DNA molecule consists of two spirally arranged chains in which each unit consists of a sugar (deoxyribose), a phosphate group and a nitrogenous base. The base can be Adenine, Guanine, Thymine or Cytosine (A,G,T or C).

A gene is a segment of DNA that carries a genetic message. One gene carries instructions for the synthesis of one protein or enzyme. Enzymes are the functioning units of the cell.

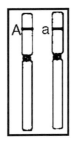

Fig. **The Genes are Situated on the Chromosomes.**

A locus is the point on a chromosome at which a gene is situated. Genes occur in pairs that occupy corresponding loci on a pair of chromosomes.

The genes at a locus are called alleles.

An individual is homozygous if the two alleles are identical e.g. AA or aa.

An individual is heterozygous if the two alleles are different e.g. Aa.

A A	*A a*	*a a*
Homozygous	*Heterozygous*	*Homozygous*

The genotype of an individual indicates the type of alleles present (heterozygous or homozygous).

The phenotype of an individual indicates the identifiable characteristics present in an individual. These may be visible or biochemical characteristics. Examples of phenotypic characteristics are eye colour, height, blood group.

A dominant characteristic is one that manifests itself in heterozygotes (i.e. only one gene is required for its manifestation in the phenotype). A recessive characteristic is one that appears only in homozygotes (i.e. two identical alleles are required for its manifestation in the phenotype).

An X-linked gene is one that is situated on the X chromosome. An X-linked recessive characteristic is usually manifest in males while females are carriers of the gene. An X-linked dominant characteristic is manifest in both sexes. The following is an example of an inherited trait for brown or blue eyes.

Alleles	B - gene for brown eyes b - gene for blue eyes		
Genotype	B B Homozygote	B b Heterozygote	b b Homozygote
Phenotype	Brown eyes	Brown eyes	Blue eyes

"Brown eyes" is the dominant characteristic because it appears in the heterozygote (Bb). "Blue eyes" is the recessive characteristic because it appears only in the homozygote (bb).

It is possible to work out how genes are inherited by constructing a Punnett square. In this example both parents were heterozygous. The phenotypes of the offspring were 3 brown: 1 blue eyes. The genotypes of the offspring were 1 dominant homozygote (BB): 2 heterozygote: 1 recessive homozygote (bb)

The inheritance of the phenotype can be illustrated as a pedigree. The following pedigree shows inheritance of eye colour.

The arrow indicates the propositus or proband i.e. the individual with a particular characteristic through whom the family came to be investigated. In this case the propositus was a boy with blue eyes.

EMERGENCE OF THE SCIENCE OF GENETICS

Mendel published his findings in 1866, but they went largely unnoticed for more than three decades. In the year 1900, however, Dutch botanist Hugo Marie de Vries, German botanist Karl Correns, and Austrian botanist Erich Tschermak independently rediscovered the monk's works and verified his conclusions. Advances in cytology, the science of the structure and function of cells, enabled scientists to more deeply appreciate Mendel's work. In 1902 American biologist Walter S. Sutton and German cell biologist Theodor Boveri separately noted the parallels between Mendel's units and chromosomes.

The demonstration of the chromosomal basis of inheritance gave rise to the modern science of genetics. The term *genetics* itself was coined in 1905 by British biologist William Bateson. The terms *gene* and *genotype* were contributed in 1909 by German scientist Wilhelm Johannsen.

In 1905 American biologists Edmund B. Wilson and Nettie Stevens independently discovered and identified the sex chromosomes. Wilson discovered the X chromosome in a butterfly, and Stevens discovered the Y chromosome in a beetle. The discoveries of the X and Y chromosomes helped scientists begin to unravel new patterns of inheritance. Foremost among this research was the work of American biologist Thomas Hunt Morgan on fruit flies. In 1910 Morgan identified the first proof of a sex-linked trait, an eye-colour characteristic that resides on the X chromosome of fruit flies. With this finding, Morgan became the first scientist to pin down the location of a gene to a specific chromosome. Morgan was also the first to explain the implications of linkage, unusual patterns of inheritance that occur when multiple genes found on the same chromosome are inherited together.

A student of Morgan's, American biologist Alfred Sturtevant, found early evidence of the mechanisms of crossing over, the phenomenon in which chromosomes interchange genes. More definitive proof emerged in the 1930s with work by American geneticists Harriet Creighton and Barbara McClintock. The pair demonstrated gene recombination with experiments on seed colour in corn. McClintock later gained notice for her work on transposable elements, large genetic segments that move within a chromosome or even between chromosomes. Her research into these elements, commonly known as jumping genes, earned McClintock the 1983 Nobel Prize in physiology or medicine.

Breakthroughs in DNA Studies

While cytologists and geneticists were studying the properties and location of genes on chromosomes, other scientists focused their studies on the composition of genes. In 1928 British microbiologist Frederick Griffith ran a series of experiments on two strains of bacteria, one that kills mice and another that is harmless to them. When Griffith injected mice with killed cells of the virulent bacteria, all of the mice survived. But in a second trial, when Griffith injected a combined cocktail of dead virulent bacteria and live "harmless" bacteria, the mice all died. He concluded that something in the dead virulent cells "transformed" the hereditary material of normally harmless bacteria so that they became killers. Most scientists at the time theorized that the transforming factor was composed of a protein.

The real identity of the transforming factor in this experiment was not identified until 1944, when American geneticists Oswald Avery, Colin MacLeod, and Maclyn McCarty revisited Griffith's research. After isolating different molecular components from dead bacterial cells, Avery and his colleagues determined that DNA was the agent that transformed the live harmless bacteria into killers.

Despite a growing body of evidence about the function of DNA, many scientists were not ready to reject proteins as the hereditary material. The debate was largely quieted in 1952 by American geneticists Alfred Hershey and Martha Chase. Hershey and Chase showed that when a type of virus called a bacteriophage infects a bacterium, it is the virus's DNA —not protein— that enters the bacterium to cause infection. Their studies confirmed that DNA contained the virus's genetic information, which triggered viral replication within the bacteria.

The experiments of Hershey and Chase convinced most scientists that DNA was the molecule of heredity, but many questions about the structure and mechanisms of DNA remained.

In the early 1950s researchers began to apply techniques of X-ray diffraction to learn about the basic structure of DNA. X-ray diffraction can determine molecular structures by measuring patterns of scattered X rays after they pass through a crystalline substance. British physical chemist Rosalind Franklin and British biophysicist Maurice Wilkins used X-ray diffraction to obtain DNA images of unprecedented clarity.

Yet the exact three-dimensional structure of DNA remained unclear. The groundbreaking work of American biochemist James Watson and British biophysicist Francis Crick solved that mystery. In 1953 the two proposed a model of DNA that is still accepted today: A double helix molecule formed by two chains, each composed of alternating sugar and phosphate groups, connected by nitrogenous bases. Watson and Crick (along with Wilkins) were awarded the 1962 Nobel Prize in physiology or medicine for their discoveries.

Watson and Crick speculated that the structure of DNA provided some obvious clues about how the molecule could replicate itself. They proposed a replication model in which each strand of DNA serves as a template for making exact copies. This model of replication, called semi-conservative replication, was demonstrated in 1958 by American molecular biologists Matthew Meselson and Franklin Stahl. Their experiments demonstrated the mechanisms of replication by tracking DNA containing a heavy nitrogen isotope through a series of replications.

With DNA's structure and replication mechanisms largely solved, scientists turned their attention to identifying the genetic code—learning how a gene's nucleotide sequence determines what type of protein is made. In the late 1950s, South African geneticist Sydney Brenner and other scientists confirmed that RNA acted as an intermediary between DNA and protein production. Researchers still were uncertain how the sequence of nucleotides in DNA corresponded to the production of specific amino acids. In 1961 Crick and Brenner determined that groups of three nucleotides, now known as codons, code for the 20 amino acids that form the foundation of proteins. The exact relationship between codons and amino acids was clarified after several important discoveries.

American biochemists Marshall Nirenberg and J. Heinrich Matthaei synthesized repeated nucleotide sequences that led to the production of repeated single amino acids. They identified how certain codon combinations code for a specific amino acid. A process developed by American geneticist Har Gobind Khorana helped scientists create a "dictionary" of codons that defined specific amino acids, thus resolving the remaining ambiguities in the genetic code. Only 12 years after the structure of DNA was deduced, the genetic code was solved.

Leharning to Manipulate DNA

After scientists had unravelled the structure and replication mechanisms of DNA, many felt that the major discoveries of genetic research were resolved. They predicted that the only task left in genetics was to sort out the molecular details of how genes work.

But in the process of studying gene function, researchers developed powerful new molecular techniques, enabling them to analyse and manipulate genes with a speed and precision never before possible.

A number of discoveries made during the 1960s and 1970s shed light on how distinct fragments of DNA could be isolated. The work of Swiss molecular biologist Werner Arber focused on specialized enzymes that digest, or "restrict," the DNA of viruses infecting bacteria. These enzymes were subsequently dubbed restriction enzymes. In the following decade, scientists learned that restriction enzymes could also act like molecular scissors to cut DNA. In 1970 American molecular biologist Hamilton Smith and colleagues determined that restriction enzymes could cleave DNA molecules at precise and predictable locations. Hamilton concluded that the enzymes were able to recognize specific nucleotide sequences.

Scientists quickly realized that restriction enzymes could be used in the laboratory to manipulate DNA. In 1973 American biochemist Herb Boyer used restriction enzymes to produce a DNA molecule with genetic material from two different sources. This splicing technique is now known as recombinant DNA. Boyer inserted foreign genes into plasmids and observed that the plasmids could replicate to make many copies of the inserted genes. In subsequent experiments, Boyer, American biochemist Stanley Cohen, and other researchers demonstrated that inserting a recombinant DNA molecule into a host bacteria cell would lead to extremely rapid replication and the production of many identical copies of the recombinant DNA. This process, known as cloning, gave scientists the power to make many copies of desired DNA for molecular study.

The speed and efficiency of DNA cloning were vastly improved in the 1980s with the invention of polymerase chain reaction (PCR). Developed by

American biochemist Kary Mullis, PCR enables scientists to produce large amounts of DNA sequences in a test tube. In a matter of hours, the process can produce millions of cloned DNA molecules. Yet all of the advances in isolating and replicating DNA would not be possible or be of much use if researchers could not determine the nucleotide sequence of genetic material. In the late 1970s and early 1980s, British biochemist Frederick Sanger and his associates developed DNA sequencing techniques.

Sanger's methods, which used special compounds called dideoxy nucleotides, rapidly yielded the exact nucleotide sequence of a desired sample. With the use of automated equipment, the new techniques transformed genetic sequencing into a speedy, routine laboratory procedure.

Many of the new techniques for isolating, sequencing, and replicating DNA have been put to practical use through the field of genetic engineering. The Human Genome Project and the new field of proteomics have both benefited from continuing technical advances and have accelerated the development of new genetic technologies. Modern genetics is poised to radically change the practice of medicine and the biotechnology industry.

THE GENETIC CODE

The structure of DNA encodes all the information every cell needs to function and thrive. In addition, DNA carries hereditary information in a form that can be copied and passed intact from generation to generation. A gene is a segment of DNA.

The biochemical instructions found within most genes, known as the genetic code, specify the chemical structure of a particular protein. Proteins are composed of long chains of amino acids, and the specific sequence of these amino acids dictates the function of each protein. The DNA structure of a gene determines the arrangement of amino acids in a protein, ultimately determining the type and function of the protein manufactured.

DNA Structure

DNA molecules form from chains of building blocks called nucleotides. Each nucleotide consists of a sugar molecule called deoxyribose that bonds to a phosphate molecule and to a nitrogen-containing compound, known as a base. DNA uses four bases in its structure: adenine (A), cytosine (C), guanine (G), and thymine (T). The order of the bases in a DNA molecule— the genetic code—determines the amino acid sequence of a protein.

In the cells of most organisms, two long strands of DNA join in a single molecule that resembles a spiralling ladder, commonly called a double helix. Alternating phosphate and sugar molecules form each side of this ladder. Bases from one DNA strand join with bases from another strand to form the rungs of the ladder, holding the double helix together.

The pairing of bases in the DNA double helix is highly specific—adenine always joins with thymine, and guanine always links to cytosine. These base combinations, known as complementary base pairing, play a fundamental role in DNA's function by aiding in the replication and storage of genetic information. Complementary base pairing also enables scientists to predict the sequence of bases on one strand of a DNA molecule if they know the order on the corresponding, or complementary, DNA strand. Scientists use complementary base pairing to help identify the genes on a particular chromosome and to develop methods used in genetic engineering.

Genes line up in a row along the length of a DNA molecule. In humans a single gene can vary in length from 100 to over 1,000,000 bases. Genes make up less than 2 per cent of the length of a DNA molecule. The rest of the DNA molecule is made up of long, highly repetitive nucleotide sequences. Once dismissed as "junk" DNA, scientists now believe these nucleotide sequences may play a role in the survival of cells. Identifying the function of these sequences is a thriving field of genetics research.

DNA Replication

In order for inherited traits to be transmitted from parent to child, the genetic information encoded in DNA must be copied with great precision during cell division. The accuracy of DNA replication depends upon the complementary pairing of bases. During replication, the DNA double helix unwinds and bonds joining the base pairs break, separating the DNA molecule into two separate strands. Each strand of DNA directs the synthesis of another complementary strand. The unpaired bases of each DNA strand attach to bases floating within the cell. But the DNA strand's unpaired bases bond only with specific, complementary bases—for example, an adenine base will bond only with a thymine base and a cytosine bases will pair only with a guanine base.

Once all of the bases of a DNA strand bond to complementary bases, the complementary bases then link to each other, forming a new DNA double-helix molecule. Thus the original DNA molecule replicates into two DNA molecules that are exact duplicates.

Gene Regulation

The processes that enable information to be copied from genes and then used to synthesize proteins must be regulated if an organism is to survive. Different cells within an organism share the same set of chromosomes. In each cell some genes are active while others are not.

For example, in humans only red blood cells manufacture the protein hemoglobin and only pancreas cells make the digestive enzyme known as trypsin, even though both types of cells contain the genes to produce both hemoglobin and trypsin. Each cell produces different proteins according to its needs so that it does not waste energy by producing proteins that will not be used.

A variety of mechanisms regulate gene activity in cells. One method involves turning on or off gene transcription, sometimes by blocking the action of RNA polymerase, an enzyme that initiates transcription. Gene regulation may also involve mechanisms that slow or speed the rate of transcription, using specialized regulatory proteins that bind to DNA. Depending on an organism's particular needs, one regulatory protein may spur transcription for a particular protein, and later, another regulatory protein may slow or halt transcription.

Prokaryotes

The bacterium *Escherichia coli* (commonly referred to as *E. coli*), found in the intestines of humans and other mammals, provides a good example of gene regulation. *E. coli* uses three enzymes to digest lactose, the primary sugar found in milk. The bacterium produces great quantities of lactose-digesting enzymes when lactose is present and saves energy by not synthesizing the enzymes when the sugar is not available. *E. coli* prefers consuming glucose to lactose, so the bacterium produces these enzymes in the presence of lactose only when no glucose is available. A region of DNA known as an operon controls this gene regulation process. In *E. coli*, the operon includes at least five genes: Three genes, called lac genes, code for the enzymes that digest lactose; one gene encodes for a regulatory protein, called a repressor, that can sense the presence or absence of lactose; and one gene, called an operator, activates transcription, the first step in the synthesis of the lactose-digesting enzymes. In the absence of lactose, the repressor protein binds with the operator gene to block transcription. This prevents the lac genes from being transcribed and halts production of the lactose-digesting enzymes. If lactose is present, the repressor protein binds to the sugar, leaving the operator gene free to trigger transcription of the lac genes. The transcription of the lac genes produces the mRNA that will direct the production of the three lactose-digesting enzymes.

Eukaryotes

Gene regulation in eukaryotes is more complex than in bacteria and other prokaryotes. Even the simplest eukaryotes have far more genes than prokaryotes, and these genes must be turned on or off as conditions dictate. Most multicellular organisms contain different types of cells that serve specialized functions. The cells of an animal's heart, blood, skin, liver, and muscles all contain the same genes. But in order to carry out their specific functions within the body, each cell must produce different proteins and respond to changing environmental stimuli, such as glucose levels in the blood or body temperature. Such specialization is possible only with sophisticated gene regulation.

Eukaryotes use a variety of mechanisms to ensure that each cell uses the exact proteins it needs at any given moment. In one method, eukaryotic cells use DNA sequences called enhancers to stimulate the transcription of genes located far away from the point on the chromosome where transcription occurs. If a specific protein binds to an enhancer site on the DNA, it causes the DNA to fold so that the enhancer site is brought closer to the site where transcription occurs. This action can activate or speed up transcription in the genes surrounding the enhancer site, thereby affecting the type and quantity of proteins the cell will produce. Enhancers often exert their effects on large groups of related genes, such as the genes that produce the set of proteins that form a muscle cell.

Gene regulation can also take place after transcription has occurred by interfering with the steps that modify mRNA before it leaves the nucleus to take part in translation. This process typically involves removing exons (segments that code for specific proteins) and introns. These sections of the mRNA can be modified in more than one way, enabling a cell to synthesize different proteins depending on its needs.

THE TOOLS OF GENETIC ENGINEERING

Cutting and Measuring DNA

The first step in gene cloning is cutting DNA into appropriately sized pieces. The size of DNA molecules is measured by subjecting the DNA to a technique called "electrophoresis". An electrophoretic apparatus gives

DNA an electrical shove (DNA is negatively charged because of its phosphate groups. The electrophoresis apparatus puts the DNA in an electric field, and it moves towards the positive pole), forcing it to move through a porous gel. Two types of gels are commonly used.

Agarose Gels

The most popular variant of electrophoresis is carried out with agarose gels. In the laboratory, suspensions of agarose in buffer are heated to boiling (often in microwave ovens), and the hot solution is poured on plastic or glass plates to a height of a few millimeters or so. Agarose is a derivative of agar — an edible polysaccharide extracted from seaweed. When cooled from heated solutions, solutions of agarose form a nearly transparent gel that looks like a slab of gelatin dessert. After the gel sets, DNA solutions are placed in little depressions formed by leaving a comb in the gel. The gel is then flooded with a weak salt solution, and a voltage is applied. Since DNA is negatively charged (due to its phosphate groups), it moves towards the positive pole.

Large DNA molecules advance slowly in the gel because they are impeded by the gel matrix. Smaller ones encounter fewer barriers and move more quickly. By plotting the distance migrated against the reciprocal of size (in base pairs) of a group of DNA standards, a fairly straight line can be obtained. From these data, the length of unknowns can be easily calculated. For ease of comparison, the standards are usually run in the same gel beside the unknowns.

Gels of differing porosities can be made by adjusting the concentration of agarose. With 2 and 3 per cent solutions, double-stranded DNA's as small as 50 or 100 base pairs can be resolved. More dilute gels can resolve fragments as large as about 30,000 base pairs (30 kilobase pairs or 30kb).

Polyacrylamide Gels

When very small DNA molecules need to be analyzed or when high-resolution separations are required, electrophoresis is carried out in polyacrylamide gels.

They, like the gels made from agarose, are water white. Unlike agarose, polyacrylamide gels are polymers of acrylamide, a small synthetic organic compound. Polyacrylamide gel electrophoresis (PAGE) is most often used to separate fragments of DNA that are between 6 and a few thousand base pairs in length. The technique is used mostly in DNA sequencing, a topic that we'll come back to later in the course.

Detecting DNA

DNA doesn't have any colour; it only absorbs light in the ultraviolet range. How is it visualized in a clear gel after electrophoresis? DNA can be detected in both agarose and polyacrylamide gels after staining with various dyes, incuding ethidium bromide, a dye that forms a fluorescent complex upon binding to DNA. Usually, the ethidium bromide is added to the gel before electrophoresis. After the run, the gel is examined and often photographed under an ultraviolet light. Yellow-orange zones (bands) of fluorescence appear (similar to those in the picture at the right), indicating migration of discrete pieces of DNA. Other agents — like methylene blue or silver stains — can also be used to visualize DNA, but they are either less sensitive or less convient, and aren't used as often. By the way, many dyes that bind to DNA are mutagenic; *i.e*, they cause mutations.

Separating Large Fragments of DNA

Contrary to what you might expect, very large fragments of DNA readily move in agarose gels when an electrical field is applied. But they don't separate according to size. In fact, very big pieces of DNA all migrate at about the same velocity regardless of whether they are 20kb in length or 2000kb.

PFE

Since many techniques, particulary recently derived ones, depend on working with very large DNA fragments, even pieces the size of some chromosomes, several newly developed electrophoretic techniques have been developed. In one of these, called pulsed field electrophoresis (PFE), DNA molecules are analyzed on agarose gels but with a modified apparatus. Instead of having only two sets of electrodes situated at opposite ends of the electrophoresis device as in the picture shown above, the pulsed field apparatus bears four sets of electrodes. Two are designated A- and A+ and the other two are called B- and B+. The two A's and the two B's are set at an angle of 120° with respect to one another. During electrophoresis, the DNA molecules are subjected to alternating bursts of current from the two A and B pairs, thereby pulling the DNA alternately to the right and to the left as it advances (from south to north in this case) through the gel. The DNA seems to reorient itself each time the current is switched, and the time that it takes to turn itself around is dependent on its length. The result is that very large pieces of DNA can be separated from another on the basis of their size. The technique also allows one to estimate the length of an unknown when run beside standards of known size. One of the most impressive accomplishments of this technique is the separation of the 16 chromosomes of yeast in a single electrophoretic run.

FIE

Another procedure, field inversion electrophoresis, is also effective at separating large molecules of DNA. In it, the electrodes are set up as in ordinary electrophoresis, but the current is switched so that the DNA first moves forward and then backward.

Of course, if the switching were to be done in equal time intervals — say, 1 second forward and 1 second back — the DNA wouldn't move at all. To get it to move at all, electrophoresis is conducted forward for a longer time than backward (or at a greater voltage forward versus backward). One might expect that moving ahead three steps and back two would be equivalent to moving forward one step at a time, but that's not what happens.

Apparently the DNA reorients itself during the switching cycles, just as it does in pulsed field electrophoresis. Again, the ability to change directions seems to be dependent on size. This allows different lengths of DNA to be separated from one another.

Restriction Endonucleases

One critically important advance that has greatly stimulated the rapid progress in molecular biology and genetic engineering was the discovery of a set of enzymes that are capable of cutting DNA at defined sequences. These enzymes are found in a variety of microorganisms and are called restriction endonucleases, or more simply, restriction enzymes.

The first specific restriction enzyme was discovered by Hamilton Smith in 1970, an accomplishment for which he (and two others) were awarded the Nobel Prize. Since then, some 3,059 similar enzymes have been reported (as of April 6, 1999), many of which have different specificities.

Nomenclature

Smith and another Nobel laureate, Daniel Nathans, devised a nomenclature for these enzymes. In brief, the name of each restriction enzyme derives from the organism from which it is isolated. The first letter of the genus name plus the first two letters of the species name form the first three letters of the restriction enzyme's name.

If necessary, a letter indicating strain designation is added, and finally a number is appended that stands for the order in which the enzyme was discovered in each organism. For example, BamHI is the name of an enzyme that is isolated from the bacterium *Bacillus amyloliquifaciens*, strain H, and it was, presumably, the first restriction endonuclease identified from that source. The first three letters of the name should be italicized, but because italicized letters are often hard to read on a computer, I have left them in plain text throughout these notes.

What they Do

The restriction enzymes owe their usefulness to the fact that they bind to DNA at specific DNA sequences, four to eight nucleotides in size, called recognition sites.

Once bound, restriction enzymes cut the DNA at or near this site. With a little thought, it should be clear that an enzyme that has a six base pair recognition site will, on the average, produce larger pieces of DNA than one that recognizes a four base site. Expressed quantitatively, the approximate size of the fragments produced by a particular enzyme, given that it is cutting a DNA containing an equal proportion of all four nucleotides, can be calculated from the formula:

Average size of fragment = 4^N

where N is the number of bases that the enzyme recognizes. Hence, a four-cutter (the shorthand name for an enzyme that recognizes a site containing four base pairs) is expected to cleave random DNA into fragments of about 4^4 (256) base pairs while an enzyme with a recognition site of six bases will produce pieces (on the average) of about 4^6 (4096) base pairs.

Properties of restriction enzymes

Ends

Another interesting property of restriction enzymes is that while they often recognize a symmetrical site, they do not always cut at the axis of symmetry. Similarly, the enzyme BglII (from the microorganisms, *Bacillus globiggi* and universally and irreverently pronounced BAGEL TWO) recognizes the sequence AGATCT and cuts between the first A and G residues.

In fact, the four nucleotide single-stranded ends are the same for both BglII and BamHI. Moreover, there are at least two other six cutting enzymes that have been discovered that leave the same four nucleotide overhang: BclI and XhoII. These overhanging ends are very useful because — under the proper conditions — they may base pair with each other. In fact, because of their affinity for one another, they are often called cohesive or sticky ends.

Moreover, if molecules with these ends are treated with the appropriate enzyme — DNA ligase — their phosphodiester bonds may be rejoined (ligated). When two ends that originate from digestion by a single enzyme are ligated, the resulting molecule can be cut by the same enzyme again. But if the ends of a DNA molecule that originated with a BamHI cut and a BglII cut are joined together, the new sequence will not be cut with either enzyme (I'll ask you to explain why this is so in class). All restriction endonucleases do not generate 5' single-strand overhangs.

In fact, some don't even produce an overhang at all. Several enzymes — like SacI — produce 3' single-stranded sticky ends. And some enzymes — like PvuII — cut at the axis of symmetry, leaving perfectly aligned ends. DNA molecules without overhangs are said to have blunt ends.In addition there are restriction enzymes that cleave DNA some distance away from the sequence that they recognize. For example the enzyme HgaI makes staggered cuts that lie 5 and 10 nucleotides away from a 5 base pair sequence, GACGC. This leaves 5' overhanging ends, but, in contrast to the enzymes described above, these will be different almost every time the enzyme cuts.

The Utility of the Restriction Enzymes

The discovery of these many restriction endonucleases have allowed genetic engineers to cut pieces of DNA at specific sites and into defined sizes. The result has been that a scientist can work with a collection of molecules all of the same size and with ends of known sequence. Restriction enzymes have proved to be valuable analytical and diagnostic tools as well.

Restriction Enzymes

Restriction enzymes are DNA-cutting enzymes found in bacteria (and harvested from them for use). Because they cut within the molecule, they are often called restriction endonucleases. A restriction enzyme recognizes and cuts DNA only at a particular sequence of nucleotides. For example, the bacterium Hemophilus aegypticus produces an enzyme named HaeIII that cuts DNA wherever it encounters the sequence

5'GGCC3'

3'CCGG5'

The cut is made between the adjacent G and C. This particular sequence occurs at 11 places in the circular DNA molecule of the virus phiX174. Thus treatment of this DNA with the enzyme produces 11 fragments, each with a precise length and nucleotide sequence. These fragments can be separated from one another and the sequence of each determined.

HaeIII and AluI cut straight across the double helix producing "blunt" ends. However, many restriction enzymes cut in an offset fashion.

The ends of the cut have an overhanging piece of single-stranded DNA. These are called "sticky ends" because they are able to form base pairs with any DNA molecule that contains the complementary sticky end. Any other source of DNA treated with the same enzyme will produce such molecules.

Mixed together, these molecules can join with each other by the base pairing between their sticky ends. The union can be made permanent by another enzyme, DNA ligase, that forms covalent bonds along the backbone of each strand. The result is a molecule of recombinant DNA (rDNA).

The ability to produce recombinant DNA molecules has not only revolutionized the study of genetics, but has laid the foundation for much of the biotechnology industry. The availability of human insulin (for diabetics), human factor VIII (for males with hemophilia A), and other proteins used in human therapy all were made possible by recombinant DNA.

Recombinant DNA and Gene Cloning

Recombinant DNA is DNA that has been created artificially. DNA from two or more sources is incorporated into a single recombinant molecule.

Making Recombinant DNA (rDNA)

- Treat DNA from both sources with the same restriction endonuclease (BamHI in this case).
- BamHI cuts the same site on both molecules

5' GGATCC 3'

3' CCTAGG 5'

- The ends of the cut have an overhanging piece of single-stranded DNA.
- These are called "sticky ends" because they are able to base pair with any DNA molecule containing the complementary sticky end.
- In this case, both DNA preparations have complementary sticky ends and thus can pair with each other when mixed.
- DNA ligase covalently links the two into a molecule of recombinant DNA.

To be useful, the recombinant molecule must be replicated many times to provide material for analysis, sequencing, etc. Producing many identical copies of the same recombinant molecule is called cloning. Cloning can be done in vitro, by a process called the polymerase chain reaction (PCR). Here, however, we shall examine how cloning is done in vivo.

Cloning in vivo can be done in

- Unicellular microbes like E. coli
- Unicellular eukaryotes like yeast and
- in mammalian cells grown in tissue culture.

In every case, the recombinant DNA must be taken up by the cell in a form in which it can be replicated and expressed. This is achieved by incorporating the DNA in a vector. A number of viruses (both bacterial and of mammalian cells) can serve as vectors. But here let us examine an example of cloning using E. coli as the host and a plasmid as the vector.

2

Protein Synthesis

Genetics is the study of genes — what they are and how they work. Genes are units inside a cell that control how living organisms inherit features from their ancestors; for example, children usually look like their parents because they have inherited their parents' genes. Genetics tries to identify which features are inherited, and explain how these features pass from generation to generation.

In genetics, a feature of a living thing is called a "trait". Some traits are part of an organism's physical appearance; such as a person's eye-color, height or weight.

Other sorts of traits are not easily seen and include blood types or resistance to diseases. The way our genes and environment interact to produce a trait can be complicated. For example, the general design of a tiger's stripes is inherited, whereas the actual stripe pattern on an individual tiger is influenced by environmental factors that are difficult to determine.

Genes are made from a long molecule called DNA, which is copied and inherited across generations. DNA is made of simple units that line up in a particular order within this long molecule. The order of these units carries genetic information, similar to how the order of letters on a page carries information.

The language used by DNA is called the genetic code, which allows the genetic machinery to read the information in the genes in triplet sets of codons. This information is the instructions for constructing and operating a living organism.

The information within a particular gene is not always exactly the same between one organism and another, so different copies of a gene do not always give exactly the same instructions. Each unique form of a single gene is called an allele. As an example, one allele for the gene for hair color could instruct the body to produce a lot of pigment, producing black hair, while a different allele of the same gene might give garbled instructions that fail to produce any pigment, giving white hair. Mutations are random changes in genes, and can create new alleles. Mutations can also produce new traits, such as when mutations to an allele for black hair produce a new allele for white hair. This appearance of new traits is important in evolution.

INHERITANCE IN BIOLOGY

Genes and Inheritance

Genes are inherited as units, with two parents dividing out copies of their genes to their offspring. This process can be compared with mixing two hands of cards, shuffling them, and then dealing them out again. Humans have two copies of each of their genes, and make copies that are found in eggs or sperm—but they only include one copy of each type of gene. An egg and sperm join to form a complete set of genes. The eventually resulting child has the same number of genes as their parents, but for any gene one of their two copies comes from their father, and one from their mother.

The effects of this mixing depend on the types (the alleles) of the gene. If the father has two copies of an allele for red hair, and the mother has two copies for brown hair, all their children get the two alleles that give different instructions, one for red hair and one for brown. The hair color of these children depends on how these alleles work together. If one allele overrides the instructions from another, it is called the *dominant* allele, and the allele that is overridden is called the *recessive* allele. In the case of a daughter with alleles for both red and brown hair, brown is dominant and she ends up with brown hair.

Although the red color allele is still there in this brown-haired girl, it doesn't show. This is a difference between what you see on the surface (the traits of an organism, called its phenotype) and the genes within the organism (its genotype). In this example you can call the allele for brown "B" and the allele for red "b". (It is normal to write dominant alleles with capital letters and recessive ones with lower-case letters.)

The brown hair daughter has the "brown hair phenotype" but her genotype is Bb, with one copy of the B allele, and one of the b allele. Now imagine that this woman grows up and has children with a brown hair man who also has a Bb genotype. Her eggs will be a mixture of two types, one sort containing the B allele, and one sort the b allele. Similarly, her partner will produce a mix of two types of sperm containing one or the other of these two alleles. When the transmitted genes are joined up in their offspring, these children have a chance of getting either brown or red hair, since they could get a genotype of BB = brown hair, Bb = brown hair or bb = red hair. In this generation, there is therefore a chance of the recessive allele showing itself in the phenotype of the children - some of them may have red hair like their grandfather.

Many traits are inherited in a more complicated way than the example above. This can happen when there are several genes involved, each contributing a small part to the end result. Tall people tend to have tall children because their children get a package of many alleles that each contribute a bit to how much they grow.

However, there are not clear groups of "short people" and "tall people", like there are groups of people with brown or red hair. This is because of the large number of genes involved; this makes the trait very variable and people are of many different heights. Despite a common misconception, the green/blue eye traits are also inherited in this complex inheritance model. Inheritance can also be complicated when the trait depends on interaction between genetics and environment. For example, malnutrition does not change traits like eye color, but can stunt growth.

Inherited Diseases

Some diseases are hereditary and run in families; others, such as infectious diseases, are caused by the environment. Other diseases come from a combination of genes and the environment. Genetic disorders are diseases that are caused by a single allele of a gene and are inherited in families. These include Huntington's disease, Cystic fibrosis or Duchenne muscular dystrophy. Cystic fibrosis, for example, is caused by mutations in a single gene called *CFTR* and is inherited as a recessive trait. Other diseases are influenced by genetics, but the genes a person gets from their parents only change their risk of getting a disease. Most of these diseases are inherited in a complex way, with either multiple genes involved, or coming from both genes and the environment.

As an example, the risk of breast cancer is 50 times higher in the families most at risk, compared to the families least at risk. This variation is probably due to a large number of alleles, each changing the risk a little bit. Several of the genes have been identified, such as *BRCA1* and *BRCA2*, but not all of them. However, although some of the risk is genetic, the risk of this cancer is also increased by being overweight, drinking a lot of alcohol and not exercising. A woman's risk of breast cancer therefore comes from a large number of alleles interacting with her environment, so it is very hard to predict.

How Genes Work

Genes Make Proteins

The function of genes is to provide the information needed to make molecules called proteins in cells. Cells are the smallest independent parts of organisms: the human body contains about 100 trillion cells, while very small organisms like bacteria are just one single cell. A cell is like a miniature and very complex factory that can make all the parts needed to produce a copy of itself, which happens when cells divide. There is a simple division of labor in cells - genes give instructions and proteins carry out these instructions, tasks like building a new copy of a cell, or repairing damage.

Each type of protein is a specialist that only does one job, so if a cell needs to do something new, it must make a new protein to do this job. Similarly, if a cell needs to do something faster or slower than before, it makes more or less of the protein responsible. Genes tell cells what to do by telling them which proteins to make and in what amounts.

Proteins are made of a chain of 20 different types of amino acid molecules. This chain folds up into a compact shape, rather like an untidy ball of string. The shape of the protein is determined by the sequence of amino acids along its chain and it is this shape that, in turn, determines what the protein does. For example, some proteins have parts of their surface that perfectly match the shape of another molecule, allowing the protein to bind to this molecule very tightly. Other proteins are enzymes, which are like tiny machines that alter other molecules.

The information in DNA is held in the sequence of the repeating units along the DNA chain. These units are four types of nucleotides (A,T,G and C) and the sequence of nucleotides stores information in an alphabet called the genetic code. When a gene is read by a cell the DNA sequence is copied into a very similar molecule called RNA (this process is called transcription). Transcription is controlled by other DNA sequences (such as promoters), which show a cell where genes are, and control how often they are copied. The RNA copy made from a gene is then fed through a structure called a ribosome, which translates the sequence of nucleotides in the RNA into the correct sequence of amino acids and joins these amino acids together to make a complete protein chain. The new protein then folds up into its active form. The process of moving information from the language of RNA into the language of amino acids is called translation.

If the sequence of the nucleotides in a gene changes, the sequence of the amino acids in the protein it produces may also change - if part of a gene is deleted, the protein produced is shorter and may not work any more. This is the reason why different alleles of a gene can have different effects in an organism. As an example, hair color depends on how much of a dark substance called melanin is put into the hair as it grows. If a person has a normal set of the genes involved in making melanin, they make all the proteins needed and they grow dark hair. However, if the alleles for a particular protein have different sequences and produce proteins that can't do their jobs, no melanin is produced and the person has white skin and hair (albinism).

Genes are Copied

Genes are copied each time a cell divides into two new cells. The process that copies DNA is called DNA replication. It is through a similar process that a child inherits genes from its parents, when a copy from the mother is mixed with a copy from the father. DNA can be copied very easily and accurately because each piece of DNA can direct the creation of a new copy of its information. This is because DNA is made of two strands that pair together like the two sides of a zipper. The nucleotides are in the center, like the teeth in the zipper, and pair up to hold the two strands together. Importantly, the four different sorts of nucleotides are different shapes, so for the strands to close up properly, an A nucleotide must go opposite a T nucleotide, and a G opposite a C. This exact pairing is called base pairing.

When DNA is copied, the two strands of the old DNA are pulled apart by enzymes that move along each of the two single strands pairing up new nucleotide units and then zipping the strands closed. This produces two new pieces of DNA, each containing one strand from the old DNA and one newly made strand. This process isn't perfect and sometimes the proteins make mistakes and put the wrong nucleotide into the strand they are building. This causes a change in the sequence of that gene. These changes in DNA sequence are called mutations. Mutations produce new alleles of genes. Sometimes these changes stop the gene from working properly, like the melanin genes discussed above. In other cases these mutations can change what the gene does or even let it do its job a little better than before. These mutations and their effects on the traits of organisms are one of the causes of evolution.

Genes and Evolution

A population of organisms evolves when an inherited trait becomes more common or less common over time. For instance, all the mice living on an island would be a single population of mice. If over a few generations, white mice went from being rare, to being a large part of this population, then the coat color of these mice would be evolving. In terms of genetics, this is called a change in allele frequency—such as an increase in the frequency of the allele for white fur.

Alleles become more or less common either just by chance (in a process called genetic drift), or through natural selection. In natural selection, if an allele makes it more likely for an organism to survive and reproduce, then over time this allele becomes more common. But if an allele is harmful, natural selection makes it less common. For example, if the island was getting colder each year and was covered with snow for much of the time, then the allele for white fur would become useful for the mice, since it would make them harder to see against the snow. Fewer of the white mice would be eaten by predators, so over time white mice would out-compete mice with dark fur. White fur alleles would become more common, and dark fur alleles would become more rare.

Mutations create new alleles. These alleles have new DNA sequences and can produce proteins with new properties. So if an island was populated entirely by black mice, mutations could happen creating alleles for white fur. The combination of mutations creating new alleles at random, and natural selection picking out those that are useful, causes adaptation. This is when organisms change in ways that help them to survive and reproduce.

MEMBRANE PROTEINS

Transmembrane proteins

G-protein-Coupled Receptors

The major role of G-protein-coupled receptors is to transmit signals into the cell. They are characterized by seven transmembrane segments. This class of membrane proteins can respond to a wide range of agonists, including photon, amines, hormones, neurotransmitters and proteins. Some agonists bind to the extracellular loops of the receptor, others may penetrate into the transmembrane region.

Immunoglobulin Family

This protein family transmit signals for immune responses. Each of them contains one or two transmembrane segments. The immunoglobulin (i.e., antibody) consists of four peptide chains: two heavy chains and two light chains. V_H and C_H represent the variable and conserved domains of the heavy chain, respectively; V_L and C_L denote those for the light chain. Variable domains are the binding site of antigens. To send signals into the cell, this class of proteins are typically coupled to non-receptor protein tyrosine kinase located on the cytosolic face of the plasma membrane.

Transport Proteins

According to the Transport Commission (TC) system, all transport proteins may be divided into the following classes:

a. Channels/Pores

Examples: ion channels, porins

b. Electrochemical Potential-driven transporters

Examples: uniporters, symporters and antiporters

c. Primary Active Transporters

Examples: Na^+-K^+ ATPase, H^+ ATPase, ABC Transporter Superfamily and CFTR channel.

d. Group Translocators

e. Transport Electron Carriers

f. Auxiliary Transport Proteins

g. Incompletely Characterized

Channels/Pores

Ion Channels [I]

Ion channels are a special class of proteins that conduct small ions such as Na^+, K^+, Ca^{2+} or Cl^-. The opening and closing of ion channels may depend on membrane voltage or the binding of molecules (the ligand). Its mechanism remains unclear. However, the mystery of their selectivity has been solved.

Ion Selectivity

Potassium Channels

By definition, a potassium channel conducts mainly K^+ ions while excluding Na^+ and Ca^{2+} ions. We note that a Na^+ ion is smaller than a K^+ ion. How could a channel conduct K^+ ions while excluding smaller ions? The answer lies in the ion's hydration energy.

The diameter of the potassium channel's selectivity filter (the narrowest region of its channel pore) should be about the same as the size of a Cs^+ ion (diameter = 3.3Å) because Cs^+ is the largest ion which can barely pass through the potassium channel. In a solution, ions are surrounded by water molecules. The first hydration shell of a K^+ or Na^+ ion contains six water molecules. The diameters of unhydrated Na^+ and K^+ ions are 1.96Å and 2.66Å, respectively. The effective diameter of a water molecule in a hydrated ion is larger than 2Å. Therefore, to pass through the selectivity filter, the K^+ or Na^+ ion must remove four water molecules from its first hydration shell, leaving only two (one at the front and anther at the back). The smaller Na^+ ion requires greater dehydration energy than the K^+ ion, because its nucleus has shorter distance with surrounding water molecules and thus interacting more strongly. As a result, the Na^+ ion is harder to pass through the potassium channel than the K^+ ion. The observation that lithium (Li^+) is excluded from the potassium channel can also be explained by the same energetic consideration. Divalent cations such as Ca^{2+} should also be excluded because their dehydration energies are much higher than monovalent cations.

Sodium Channels

In the sodium channel, the Na^+ ion is more permeable than the K^+ ion. This is because the selectivity filter of the sodium channel is slightly larger than that of the potassium channel. It is large enough to accommodate a Na^+ ion attached with three water molecules, but not enough for a K^+ ion attached with three water molecules. Therefore, to pass through the sodium channel, the Na^+ ion needs to remove only three, but the K^+ ion has to remove four, water molecules from its first hydration shell. The required dehydration energy for the K^+ ion is greater than the Na^+ ion.

Calcium Channels

In calcium channels, the permeability of monovalent cations (Na^+ and K^+) is about three orders of magnitude smaller than the Ca^{2+} permeability. This ion selectivity does not seem to involve hydration, because Ca^{2+} is more heavily hydrated than Na^+, and the unhydrated diameters of Ca^{2+} and Na^+ are almost identical. Then, how could calcium channels select Ca^{2+} over Na^+?

Although the permeability of monovalent cations in the calcium channel is quite small at normal ionic concentrations, large monovalent cationic current can be observed in the absence of Ca^{2+} and other divalent cations. This suggests that the calcium channel is basically permeable to both divalent and monovalent cations, but the selectivity arises from competition between ions. The calcium channel may contain a negatively charged binding site to facilitate ion conduction. The monovalent cations simply cannot compete with

Ca^{2+} for this binding site. This idea has been demonstrated experimentally. In the calcium channel, if a negatively charged glutamate residue in the pore-lining region is mutated into a positively charged lysine, the calcium channel becomes more permeable to Na^+ than Ba^{2+}. Conversely, in the sodium channel, mutation of a pore-lining lysine residue into glutamate transforms the channel from a Na^+-selective to a Ca^{2+}-selective channel.

Channel Structures

The detailed 3D structures of most ion channels are not known. However, from the hydrophobicity profile of their amino acid sequences, it is possible to obtain the domain structures of most ion channels.

K Channels

There are many types of potassium channels. Most commonly observed K channels are composed of four subunits, each is homologous to the Shaker protein. The hydrophobicity profile indicates that it contains six hydrophobic segments, designated as S1 - S6. These segments are likely to be the transmembrane domains. Other experimental results suggests that the P-region is lining the channel pore.

Na and Ca Channels

A Na or Ca channel consists of a major pore-forming subunit and possibly other small auxiliary subunits. The major pore-forming subunit is called the α subunit which can be divided into four similar domains. Each domain is analogous to a Shaker protein with six transmembrane segments and a P-region. Thus, an α subunit is sufficient to form an ion channel.

Synaptic Channels

A large class of ion channels are specifically located at the synapses (the junction between nerve cells).

Porin

The nonpolar interior of membranes limits the free diffusion of polar molecules. In most membranes various proteins serve as channels and pumps which regulate the movement of ions, metabolites and even water across the membrane. Due to the specificity of these proteins there is a high degree of control over what passes through the membrane.Several membranes such as the outer membranes of mitochondria, chloroplasts and bacteria, however, do not need the same high degree of control over what gets across. Rather than synthesizing many selective proteins to carry polar molecules across, it appears that cells make only a few types of transporters, like the porin pictured below, which let almost anything below a certain size across. It may simply be more cost effective to put a few porins in these membranes then many more selective proteins. These "leaky" membranes are still effective barriers to the movement of large molecules such as proteins.

Below are two views of a model of porin from the bacterium *Rhodopseudomonas blastica.* In the left image the model is shown from the side as if you are in the middle of the membrane. The height of the protein is about the same as the thickness of the membrane in which it sits. The right image shows the model from the end where the central "hole" through which ions and metabolites pass is clearly visible. Regions of secondary structure are shown in yellow (beta sheet), pink (alpha helix) and blue (turn). The strands of colour follow the backbone of the molecule. If all of the atoms and bonds in the protein were visualized the image would be much too complicated.Why is the tertiary structure of porin described as a beta barrel?

Electrochemical Potential-driven Transporters

Uniporter-Catalyzed Transport

We begin our discussion of membrane transport proteins with the simplest type, which catalyze uniport transport. The plasma membrane of most cells contains several uniporters that enable amino acids, nucleosides, sugars, and other small molecules to enter and leave cells down their concentration gradients. Similar to enzymes, uniporters accelerate a reaction that is already thermodynamically favored, and the movement of a substance across a membrane down its concentration gradient will have the same negative ΔG value whether or not a protein transporter is involved. This type of movement sometimes is referred to as facilitated transport (or facilitated diffusion). Many chemical reactions that are thermodynamically favored will not occur unless an appropriate enzyme is present; such is also the case with movement of hydrophilic molecules across biological membranes. Unlike the substrates of enzymatic reactions, however, transported substances undergo no chemical change during movement across a membrane.

Three Main Features Distinguish Uniport Transport from Passive Diffusion

Three properties of uniporter-catalyzed movement of glucose and other small hydrophilic molecules across a membrane distinguish this type of transport from passive diffusion:

1. The rate of facilitated transport by uniporters is far higher than predicted by Fick's equation describing passive diffusion. Because the transported molecules never enter the hydrophobic core of the phospholipid bilayer, the partition coefficient K is irrelevant.

2. Transport is specific. Each uniporter transports only a single species of molecule or a single group of closely related molecules.

3. Transport occurs via a limited number of uniporter molecules, rather *than throughout the phospholipid bilayer.* Consequently, there is a maximum transport rate V_{max} that is achieved when the concentration gradient across the membrane is very large and each uniporter is working at its maximal rate.

Cotransport by Symporters and Antiporters

Besides ATP-powered pumps, cells have a second, discrete class of proteins that import or export ions and small molecules, such as glucose and amino acids, against a concentration gradient. These proteins use the energy stored in the electrochemical gradient of Na^+ or H^+ ions to power the uphill movement of another substance, a process called cotransport. For instance, the energetically favored movement of a Na^+ ion (the "cotransported" ion) into a cell across the plasma membrane, driven both by its concentration gradient and by the transmembrane voltage gradient can be coupled obligatorily to movement of the "transported" molecule (e.g., glucose) against its concentration gradient. When the transported molecule and cotransported ion move in the same direction, the process is called symport; when they move in opposite directions, the process is called antiport.

Primary Active Transporters

Active Transport by ATP-Powered Pumps

We turn now to the ATP-powered pumps that transport ions and various small molecules against their concentration gradients. The general structures of the four principal classes of these transport proteins are depicted in figure and their properties are summarized in table. Note that the P, F, and V classes transport ions only, whereas the ABC superfamily class transports small molecules as well as ions.

P-class ion pumps containa transmembrane catalytic á subunit, which contains an ATP-binding site, and usually a smaller β subunit, which may have regulatory functions. Many of these pumps are tetramers composed of twoα and two β subunits. During the transport process, at least one of the á subunits is phosphorylated (hence the label "P"), and the transported ions are thought to move through the phosphorylated subunit. This class includes the Na^+/K^+ ATPase in the plasma membrane, which maintains the Na^+ and K^+ gradients typical of animal cells, and several Ca^{2+} ATPases, which pump Ca^{2+} ions out of the cytosol into the external medium or into the lumen of the sarcoplasmic reticulum (SR) of muscle cells. Another member of the P class, found in acid-secreting cells of the mammalian stomach, transports protons (H^+ ions) out of and K^+ ions into the cell. The H^+ pump that maintains the membrane electric potential in plant, fungal, and bacterial cells also belongs to this class.

The structures of *F-class* and *V-class ion pumps* are similar to each other but unrelated to and more complicated than P-class pumps. F- and V-class pumps contain at least three kinds of transmembrane proteins and five kinds of extrinsic polypeptides that form the cytosolic domain. Several of the transmembrane and extrinsic subunits in F-class and V-class pumps exhibit sequence homology, and each pair of homologous subunits is thought to have evolved from a common polypeptide.

All known V and F pumps transport only protons in a process that does not involve a phosphoprotein intermediate. V-class pumps generally function to maintain the low pH of plant vacuoles and of lysosomes and other acidic vesicles in animal cells by using the energy released by ATP hydrolysis to pump protons from the cytosolic to the exoplasmic face of the membrane against the proton electrochemical gradient. F-class pumps are found in bacterial plasma membranes and in mitochondria and chloroplasts. In contrast to V pumps, they generally function to power the synthesis of ATP from ADP and P_i by movement of protons from the exoplasmic to the cytosolic face of the membrane down the proton electrochemical gradient.

The final class of ATP-powered transport proteins is larger and more diverse than the other classes. Referred to as the *ABC (ATP-binding cassette) superfamily*, this class includes more than 100 different transport proteins found in organisms ranging from bacteria to humans. Each ABC protein is specific for a single substrate or group of related substrates including ions, sugars, peptides, polysaccharides, and even proteins. All ABC transport proteins share a common organization consisting of four "core" domains: two transmembrane (T) domains, forming the passageway through which transported molecules cross the membrane, and two cytosolic ATP-binding (A) domains. In some ABC proteins, the core domains are present in four separate polypeptides; in others, the core domains are fused into one or two multidomain polypeptides.

All classes of ATP-powered pumps have one or more binding sites for ATP, and these are always on the cytosolic face of the membrane. Although these proteins are often called ATPases, they normally do not hydrolyze ATP into ADP and P_i unless ions or other molecules are simultaneously transported. Because of the tight coupling between ATP hydrolysis and transport, the energy stored in the phosphoanhydride bond is not dissipated. Thus ATP-powered transport proteins are able to collect the free energy released during ATP hydrolysis and use it to move ions or other molecules uphill against a potential or concentration gradient.

The energy expended by cells to maintain the concentration gradients of Na^+, K^+, H^+, and Ca^{2+} across the plasma and intracellular membranes is considerable. In nerve and kidney cells, for example, up to 25 percent of the ATP produced by the cell is used for ion transport; in human erythrocytes, up to 50 percent of the available ATP is used for this purpose. In cells treated with poisons that inhibit the aerobic production of ATP (e.g., 2,4-dinitrophenol), the ion concentration inside the cell gradually approaches that of the exterior environment as the ions move through plasma membrane channels down their electric and concentration gradients. Eventually treated cells die: partly because protein synthesis requires a high concentration of K^+ ions and partly because in the absence of a Na^+ gradient across the cell membrane, a cell cannot import certain nutrients such as amino acids. Studies on the effects of such poisons provided early evidence for the existence of ion pumps. In this section, we discuss in some detail examples of the P, V, and ABC classes of ATP-powered pumps.

Plasma-Membrane Ca^{2+} ATPase Exports Ca^{2+} Ions from Cells.

In order for Ca^{2+} to function in intracellular signaling, its cytosolic concentration usually must be kept below $0.1 - 0.2$ μM. (Although some cytosolic Ca^{2+} is bound to negatively charged groups, it is the concentration of *free*, unbound Ca^{2+} that is critical to its signaling function.) The plasma membranes of animal, yeast, and probably plant cells contain Ca^{2+} ATPases that transport Ca^{2+} out of the cell against its electrochemical gradient. These P-class ion pumps help maintain the concentration of free Ca^{2+} ions in the cytosol at a low level.

In addition to a catalytic subunit containing an ATP-binding site, as found in other P-class pumps, plasmamembrane Ca^{2+} ATPases also contain the Ca^{2+}-binding regulatory protein calmodulin. A rise in cytosolic Ca^{2+} induces the binding of Ca^{2+} ions to calmodulin, which triggers an allosteric activation of the Ca^{2+} ATPase; as a result, the export of Ca^{2+} ions from the cell accelerates, and the original low cytosolic concentration of free Ca^{2+} is restored rapidly.

Muscle Ca^{2+} ATPase Pumps Ca^{2+} Ions from the Cytosol into the Sarcoplasmic Reticulum.

Besides the plasma-membrane Ca^{2+} ATPase, muscle cells contain a second, different Ca^{2+} ATPase that transports Ca^{2+} from the cytosol into the lumen of the sarcoplasmic reticulum (SR), an internal organelle that concentrates and stores Ca^{2+} ions. As discussed the SR and its calcium pump (referred to as the *muscle calcium pump*) are critical in muscle contraction and relaxation: release of Ca^{2+} ions from the SR into the muscle cytosol causes contraction, and the rapid removal of Ca^{2+} ions from the cytosol by the muscle calcium pump induces relaxation.

Because the muscle calcium pump constitutes more than 80 percent of the integral protein in SR membranes, it is easily purified and characterized. Each transmembrane catalytic subunit has a molecular weight of 100,000 and transports two Ca^{2+} ions per ATP hydrolyzed. In the cytosol of muscle cells, the free Ca^{2+} concentration ranges from 10^{-7} M (resting cells) to more than 10^{-6} M (contracting cells), whereas the *total* Ca^{2+} concentration in the SR lumen can be as high as 10^{-2} M. Sites on the cytosolic surface of the muscle calcium pump have a very high affinity for Ca^{2+} ($K_m = 10^{-7}$ M), allowing the pump to transport Ca^{2+} efficiently from the cytosol into the SR against the steep concentration gradient.

The concentration of free Ca^{2+} within the sarcoplasmic reticulum is actually much less than the total concentration of 10^{-2} M. Two soluble proteins in the lumen of SR vesicles bind Ca^{2+} and serve as a reservoir for intracellular Ca^{2+}, thereby reducing the concentration of free Ca^{2+} ions in the SR vesicles, and consequently decreasing the energy needed to pump Ca^{2+} ions into them from the cytosol. The activity of the muscle Ca^{2+} ATPase is so regulated that if the free Ca^{2+} concentration in the cytosol becomes too high, the rate of calcium pumping increases until the cytosolic Ca^{2+} concentration is reduced to less than 1 µM. Thus in muscle cells, the calcium pump in the SR membrane can supplement the activity of the plasma-membrane pump, assuring that the cytosolic concentration of free Ca^{2+} remains below 1 µM.

The current model of the mechanism of action of the Ca^{2+} ATPase in the SR membrane is outlined in Figure. Coupling of ATP hydrolysis with ion pumping involves several steps that must occur in a defined order. When the protein is in one conformation, termed *E1*, two Ca^{2+} ions bind in sequence to high-affinity sites on the cytosolic surface (step 1). Then an ATP binds to its site on the cytosolic surface; in a reaction requiring that a Mg^{2+} ion be tightly complexed to the ATP, the bound ATP is hydrolyzed to ADP and the liberated phosphate is transferred to a specific aspartate residue in the protein, forming a high-energy acyl phosphate bond, denoted by E1~P (step 2). The protein then changes its conformation to E2 – P, generating two lowaffinity Ca^{2+}-binding sites on the exoplasmic surface, which faces the SR lumen; this conformational change simultaneously propels the two Ca^{2+} ions through the protein to these sites (step 3) and inactivates the high-affinity Ca^{2+}-binding sites on the cytosolic face. The Ca^{2+} ions then dissociate from the exoplasmic surface of the protein (step 4). Following this, the aspartyl-phosphate bond in E2 – P is hydrolyzed, causing E2 to revert to E1, a change that inactivates the exoplasmic-facing Ca^{2+}-binding sites and regenerates the cytosolicfacing Ca^{2+}-binding sites (step 5).

Thus phosphorylation of the muscle calcium pump by ATP favors conversion of E1 to E2, and dephosphorylation favors the conversion of E2 to E1. While only E2 – P, not E1~P, is actually hydrolyzed, the free energy of hydrolysis of the aspartyl-phosphate bond in E1~P is greater than that for E2 – P. The reduction in free energy of the aspartyl-phosphate bond in E2 – P, relative to E1~P, can be said to power the E1 E2 conformational change. The affinity of Ca^{2+} for the cytosolic-facing binding sites in E1 is a thousandfold greater than the affinity of Ca^{2+} for the exoplasmic-facing sites in E2; this difference enables the protein to transport Ca^{2+} unidirectionally from the cytosol, where it binds tightly to the pump, to the exoplasm, where it is released.

For instance, the muscle calcium pump has been isolated with phosphate linked to an aspartate residue, and spectroscopic studies have detected slight alterations in protein conformation during the E1 E2 conversion. On the basis of the protein's amino acid sequence and various biochemical studies, investigators proposed the structural model for the catalytica subunit shown in Figure. The membrane-spanninga helices are thought to form the passageway through which Ca^{2+} ions move. The bulk of the subunit consists of cytosolic globular domains that are involved in ATP binding, phosphorylation of aspartate, and energy transduction. These domains are connected by "stalks" to the membrane-embedded domain.

As noted previously, all P-class ion pumps, regardless of which ion they transport, are phosphorylated during the transport process. The amino acid sequences around the phosphorylated aspartate in the catalytica subunit are highly conserved in all proteins of this type. Thus the mechanistic model in

Figure probably is generally applicable to all these ATP-powered ion pumps. In addition, the α subunits of all the P pumps examined to date have a similar molecular weight and, as deduced from their amino acid sequences derived from cDNA clones, have a similar arrangement of transmembrane α helices. These findings strongly suggest that all these proteins evolved from a common precursor, although they now transport different ions.

Na^+/K^+ ATPase Maintains the Intracellular Na^+ and K^+ Concentrations in Animal Cells.

A second P-class ion pump that has been studied in considerable detail is the Na^+/K^+ ATPase present in the plasma membrane of all animal cells. This ion pump is a tetramer of subunit composition $α_2β_2$. (Classic Experiment 15.1 describes the discovery of this enzyme.) The β polypeptide is required for newly synthesized α subunits to fold properly in the endoplasmic reticulum but apparently is not involved directly in ion pumping.

The α subunit is a 120,000-MW nonglycosylated polypeptide whose amino acid sequence and predicted membrane structure are very similar to those of the muscle Ca^{2+} ATPase. In particular, the Na^+/K^+ ATPase has a stalk on the cytosolic face that links domains containing the ATP-binding site and the phosphorylated aspartate to the membrane-embedded domain. The overall process of transport moves three Na^+ ions out of and two K^+ ions into the cell per ATP molecule split.

Several lines of evidence indicate that the Na^+/K^+ ATPase is responsible for the coupled movement of K^+ and Na^+ into and out of the cell, respectively. For example, the drug *ouabain*, which binds to a specific region on the exoplasmic surface of the protein and specifically inhibits its ATPase activity, also prevents cells from maintaining their Na^+/K^+ balance. Any doubt that the Na^+/K^+ ATPase is responsible for ion movement was dispelled by the demonstration that the enzyme, when purified from the membrane and inserted into liposomes, propels K^+ and Na^+ transport in the presence of ATP.

The mechanism of action of the Na^+/K^+ ATPase, outlined in figure is similar to that of the muscle calcium pump, except that ions are pumped in both directions across the membrane. In its E1 conformation, the Na^+/K^+ ATPase has three high-affinity Na^+-binding sites and two low-affinity K^+-binding sites on the cytosolic-facing surface of the protein. The K_m for binding of Na^+ to these cytosolic sites is 0.6 mM, a value considerably lower than the intracellular Na^+ concentration of H"12 mM; as a result, Na^+ ions normally will fill these sites. Conversely, the affinity of the cytosolic K^+-binding sites is low enough that K^+ ions, transported inward through the protein, dissociate from E1 into the cytosol despite the high intracellular K^+ concentration. During the E1 E2 transition, the three bound Na^+ ions move outward through the protein.

Transition to the E2 conformation also generates two high-affinity K^+ sites and three low-affinity Na^+ sites on the exoplasmic face. Because the K_m for K^+ binding to these sites (0.2 mM) is considerably lower than the extracellular K^+ concentration (4 mM), these sites will fill quickly with K^+ ions. In contrast, the three Na^+ ions, transported outward through the protein, will dissociate into the extracellular medium from the low-affinity Na^+ sites on the exoplasmic surface despite the high extracellular Na^+ concentration. Similarly, during the E2 E1 transition, the two bound K^+ ions are transported inward.

V-Class H^+ ATPases Pump Protons across Lysosomal and Vacuolar MembranesAll V-class ATPases transport H^+ ions only. These proton pumps, present in the membranes of lysosomes, endosomes, and plant vacuoles, function to acidify the lumen of these organelles. The acidity of the lysosomal lumen, usually H"4.5 – 5.0, can be measured precisely in living cells by use of particles labeled with a pH-sensitive fluorescent dye. Cells phagocytose these particles and transfer them to the lysosomes. The ability of different wavelengths of visible light to excite fluorescence is highly dependent on pH, and the lysosomal pH can be calculated from the spectrum of the fluorescence emitted. Maintenance of the 100-fold or more proton gradient between the lysosomal lumen (pH H"4.5 – 5.0) and the cytosol (pH H"7.0) depends on ATP production by the cell.

The ATP-powered proton pumps in lysosomal and vacuolar membranes have been isolated, purified, and incorporated into liposomes. As illustrated in figure these V-class proton pumps contain two discrete domains: a cytosolic-facing hydrophilic domain (V_1) composed of five different polypeptides and a transmembrane domain (V_0) containing 9 – 12 copies of proteolipid c, one copy of protein b, and one copy of protein a. The subunit composition of the cytosolic domain is $a_3\beta_3\gamma\delta\epsilon$; the$\alpha$ and β subunits contain the sites where ATP binding and hydrolysis occur. Each transmembrane c subunit is thought to span the membrane two times; the c and a subunits together form the proton-conducting channel. Unlike P-class ion pumps, the V-class H^+ ATPases are not phosphorylated and dephosphorylated during proton transport.

Similar V-class ATPases are found in the plasma membrane of certain acid-secreting cells. These include osteoclasts, bone-resorbing macrophagelike cells, which bind to a bone and seal off a small segment of extracellular space between the plasma membrane and the surface of the bone. HCl secreted into this space by osteoclasts dissolves the calcium phosphate crystals that give bone its rigidity and strength.

Another example is the mitochondria-rich epithelial cells lining the toad bladder; the apical plasma membrane of these cells contain many V-class H^+ ATPases, which function to acidify the urine. As we discuss later, the membrane of plant vacuoles contains two proton pumps: a typical V-class H^+ ATPase and another one that utilizes the energy released by hydrolysis of inorganic pyrophosphate (PP_i) to pump protons into the vacuole. This PP_i-hydrolyzing proton pump, believed to be unique to plants, has an amino acid sequence different from any other ion-transporting proteins

ATP-powered proton pumps cannot acidify the lumen of an organelle (or the extracellular space) by themselves. The reason for this is that pumping of protons would rapidly cause a buildup of positive charge on the exoplasmic face of the membrane on the inside of the vesicle membrane and a corresponding buildup of negative charges on the cytosolic face. In other words, the pump would generate a voltage across the membrane, exoplasmic face positive, which would prevent movement of protons into the vesicle before a significant H^+ concentration gradient had been established. In fact, this is the way that H^+ pumps generate an insidenegative potential across plant and yeast plasma membranes. In order for an organelle lumen or an extracellular space (e.g., the outside of an osteoclast) to become acidic, movement of H^+ up its concentration gradient must be accompanied by

1. Movement of an equal number of anions in the same direction or
2. Movement of equal numbers of a different cation in the opposite direction. The first process occurs in lysosomes and plant vacuoles whose membranes contain V-class H^+ ATPases and ion channels through which accompanying anions (e.g., Cl^-) move. The second occurs in the lining of the stomach, which contains a P-class H^+/K^+ ATPase that pumps one H^+ outward and one K^+ inward.

THE ABC SUPERFAMILY TRANSPORTS A WIDE VARIETY OF SUBSTRATES

As noted earlier, all members of the very large and diverse ABC superfamily of transport proteins contain two transmembrane (T) domains and two cytosolic ATP-binding (A) domains. The T domains, each built of six membrane-spanning á helices, form the pathway through which the transported substance (substrate) crosses the membrane and determine the substrate specificity of each ABC protein. The sequence of the A domains is H"30 to 40 percent homologous in all members of this superfamily, indicating a common evolutionary origin. Some ABC proteins also contain a substrate-binding subunit or regulatory subunit.

Bacterial Plasma-Membrane Permeases

The plasma membrane of many bacteria contain numerous *permeases* that belong to the ABC superfamily. These proteins use the energy released by hydrolysis of ATP to transport specific amino acids, sugars, vitamins, or even peptides into the cell. Since bacteria frequently grow in soil or pond water where the concentration of nutrients is low, these ABC transport proteins allow the cells to concentrate amino acids and other nutrients in the cell against a substantial concentration gradient. Bacterial permeases generally are *inducible;* that is, the quantity of a transport protein in the cell membrane is regulated by both the concentration of the nutrient in the medium and the metabolic needs of the cell.

In *E. coli* histidine permease, a typical bacterial ABC protein, the two transmembrane domains and two cytosolic ATP-binding domains are formed by four separate subunits. In gram-negative bacteria such as *E. coli,* which have an outer membrane, a soluble histidine-binding protein in the periplasmic space assists in transport. This soluble protein binds histidine tightly and directs it to the T subunits, through which histidine crosses the membrane powered by ATP hydrolysis. Mutant *E. coli* cells that are defective in any of the histidine-permease subunits or the soluble binding protein are unable to transport histidine into the cell, but are able to transport other amino acids whose uptake is facilitated by other transport proteins. Such genetic analyses provide strong evidence that histidine permease and similar ABC proteins function to transport solutes into the cell.

Mammalian MDR Transport Proteins

A series of rather unexpected observations led to discovery of the first eukaryotic ABC protein. Oncologists noted that tumor cells often became simultaneously resistant to several chemotherapeutic drugs with unrelated chemical structures; similarly, cell biologists observed that cultured cells selected for resistance to one toxic substance (e.g., colchicine, a microtubule inhibitor) frequently became resistant to several other drugs, including the anticancer drug adriamycin. Subsequent studies showed that this resistance is due to enhanced expression of a *multidrug-resistance (MDR) transport protein* known as *MDR1*. In this member of the ABC superfamily, all four domains are "fused" into a single 170,000-MW protein. This protein uses the energy derived from ATP hydrolysis to*export* a large variety of drugs from the cytosol to the extracellular medium. The *Mdr1* gene is frequently amplified in multidrug-resistant cells, resulting in a large overproduction of the MDR1 protein.

Most drugs transported by MDR1 are small hydrophobic molecules, which diffuse from the culture medium across the plasma membrane into the cell. The ATP-powered export of such drugs from the cytosol by MDR1 means a much higher extracellular drug concentration is required to kill cells. That MDR1 is an ATP-powered small-molecule pump has been demonstrated with liposomes containing the purified protein. The ATPase activity of these liposomes is enhanced by different drugs in a dose-dependent manner corresponding to their ability to be transported by MDR1.

Not only does MDR1 transport a varied group of molecules, but all these substrates compete with one another for transport by MDR1. Although the mechanism of action of MDR1-assisted transport has not been definitively demonstrated, the *flippase model,* is a likely candidate. Substrates of MDR1 are primarily planar, lipid-soluble molecules with one or more positive charges, and they move spontaneously from the cytosol into the cytosolic-facing leaflet of the plasma membrane. The hydrophobic portion of a substrate molecule is oriented toward the hydrophobic core of the membrane, and the charged portion toward the polar cytosolic face of the membrane and is still in the cytosol. The substrate diffuses laterally until encountering and binding to a site on the MDR1 protein that is within the bilayer. The protein then "flips" the charged substrate molecule into the exoplasmic leaflet, an energetically unfavorable reaction powered by the coupled ATPase activity of MDR1.

Once in the exoplasmic face, the substrate diffuses into the aqueous phase on the outside of the cell. Support for the flippase model of transport by MDR1 comes from MDR2, a homologous protein present in the region of the liver cell plasma membrane that faces the bile duct. MDR2 has been shown to flip phospholipids from the cytosolic-facing leaflet of the plasma membrane to the exoplasmic leaflet, thereby generating an excess of phospholipids in the exoplasmic leaflet; these phospholipids peel off into the bile duct and form an essential part of the bile. An alternative *pump model* also has been proposed for MDR1. According to this model, drug molecules in the cytosol bind directly to a single small-molecule binding site on the cytosolic face of the MDR1 protein; subsequent ATP hydrolysis powers movement of the bound drug through the protein to the aqueous phase on the outside of the cell by a mechanism similar to that of other ATP-powered pumps.

MDR1 protein is expressed in abundance in the liver, intestines, and kidney — sites from which natural toxic products are removed from the body. Thus the natural function of MDR1 may be to transport a variety of natural and metabolic toxins into the bile, intestinal lumen, or forming urine. During the course of its evolution, MDR1 appears to have coincidentally acquired the ability to transport drugs whose structures are similar to those of these toxins. Tumors derived from these cell types, such as hepatomas (liver cancers), frequently are resistant to virtually all chemotherapeutic agents and thus difficult to treat, presumably because the tumors exhibit increased expression of the MDR1 or MDR2 proteins.

Cystic Fibrosis Transmembrane Regulator (CFTR) Protein

Discovery of another ABC transport protein came from studies of cystic fibrosis (CF), the most common lethal autosomal recessive genetic disease of Caucasians. This disease is caused by a mutation in the *CFTR* gene, which encodes a chloride-channel protein that is regulated by cyclic AMP (cAMP), an intracellular second messenger. These Cl'' channels are present in the apical plasma membranes of epithelial cells in the lung, sweat glands, pancreas, and other tissues. An increase in cAMP stimulates Cl'' transport by such cells from normal individuals, but not from CF individuals who have a defective CFTR protein.

The sequence and predicted structure of the encoded CFTR protein, based on analysis of the cloned gene, are very similar to those of MDR1 protein except for the presence of an additional domain, the regulatory (R) domain, on the cytosolic face. The Cl''-channel activity of CFTR protein clearly is enhanced by binding of ATP. Moreover, cAMP activates a protein kinase that phosphorylates, and thereby activates, CFTR. When purified CFTR protein is incorporated into liposomes, it forms Cl'' channels with properties similar to those in normal epithelial cells. And when the wild-type CFTR protein is expressed by recombinant techniques in cultured epithelial cells from CF patients, the cells recover normal Cl''-channel activity. This latter result raises the possibility that gene therapy might reverse the course of cystic fibrosis.

Since CFTR protein is similar to MDR1 in structure, it may also function as an ATP-powered pump of some as-yet unidentified molecule. In any case, much remains to be learned about this fascinating class of ABC transport proteins.

PROTEIN SYNTHESIS IN GENETICS

During the 1950s and 1960s, it became apparent that DNA is essential in the synthesis of proteins. Proteins are used in enzymes and as structural materials in cells. Many specialised proteins function in cellular activities. For example, in humans, the hormone insulin and the muscle cell filaments are composed of protein. The hair, skin, and nails of humans are composed of proteins, as are all the hundreds of thousands of enzymes in the body

The key to a protein molecule is how the amino acids are linked. The sequence of amino acids in a protein is a type of code that specifies the protein and distinguishes one protein from another. A genetic code in the DNA determines this amino acid code. The genetic code consists of the sequence of nitrogenous bases in the DNA. How the nitrogenous base code is translated to an amino acid sequence in a protein is the basis for protein synthesis.

For protein synthesis to occur, several essential materials must be present, such as a supply of the 20 amino acids, which comprise most proteins.

Another essential element is a series of enzymes that will function in the process. DNA and another form of nucleic acid called ribonucleic acid (RNA) are essential.

RNA is the nucleic acid that carries instructions from the nuclear DNA into the cytoplasm, where protein is synthesised. RNA is similar to DNA, with two exceptions. First, the carbohydrate in RNA is ribose rather than deoxyribose, and second, RNA nucleotides contain the pyrimidine uracil rather than thymine.

GENETIC ENGINEERING

Since traits come from the genes in a cell, putting a new piece of DNA into a cell can produce a new trait. This is how genetic engineering works. For example, rice can be given genes from a maize and a soil bacteria so the rice produces beta-carotene, which the body converts to Vitamin A. This can help children suffering from Vitamin A deficiency. Other genes that can be put into crops include a natural insecticide from the bacteria *Bacillus thuringiensis*. The insecticide kills insects that eat the plants, but is harmless to people. In these plants, the new genes are put into the plant before it is grown, so the genes are in every part of the plant, including its seeds. The plant's offspring inherit the new genes, which has led to concern about the spread of new traits into wild plants.

The kind of technology used in genetic engineering is also being developed to treat people with genetic disorders in an experimental medical technique called gene therapy. However, here the new gene is put in after the person has grown up and become ill, so any new gene is not inherited by their children. Gene therapy works by trying to replace the allele that causes the disease with an allele that works properly.

Principles of Genetics

Mendel's studies have provided scientists with the basis for mathematically predicting the probabilities of genotypes and phenotypes in the offspring of a genetic cross. But not all genetic observations can be explained and predicted based on Mendelian genetics. Other complex and distinct genetic phenomena may also occur. Several complex genetic concepts, described in this section, explain such distinct genetic phenomena as blood types and skin colour.

Incomplete Dominance

In some allele combinations, dominance does not exist. Instead, the two characteristics blend. In such a situation, both alleles have the opportunity to express themselves. For instance, snapdragon flowers display incomplete dominance in their colour. There are two alleles for flower colour: one for white and one for red. When two alleles for white are present, the plant displays white flowers. When two alleles for red are present, the plant has red flowers. But when one allele for red is present with one allele for white, the colour of the snapdragons is pink.

However, if two pink snapdragons are crossed, the phenotype ratio of the offspring is one red, two pink, and one white. These results show that the genes themselves remain independent; only the expressions of the genes blend. If the gene for red and the gene for white actually blended, pure red and pure white snapdragons could not appear in the offspring.

Multiple Alleles

In certain cases, more than two alleles exist for a particular characteristic. Even though an individual has only two alleles, additional alleles may be present in the population. This condition is multiple alleles.

An example of multiple alleles occurs in blood type. In humans, blood groups are determined by a single gene with three possible alleles: A, B, or O. Red blood cells can contain two antigens, A and B. The presence or absence of these antigens results in four blood types: A, B, AB, and O. If a person's red blood cells have antigen A, the blood type is A. If a person's red blood cells have antigen B, the blood type is B. If the red blood cells have both antigen A and antigen B, the blood type is AB. If the red blood cells have neither antigen A nor antigen B, the blood type is O.

The alleles for type A and type B blood are co-dominant; that is, both alleles are expressed. However, the allele for type O blood is recessive to both type A and type B. Because a person has only two of the three alleles, the blood type varies depending on which two alleles are present. For instance, if a person has the A allele and the B allele, the blood type is AB. If a person has two A alleles, or one A and one O allele, the blood type is A. If a person has two B alleles or one B and one O allele, the blood type is B. If a person has two O alleles, the blood type is O.

Polygenic Inheritance

Although many characteristics are determined by alleles at a single place on the chromosome, some characteristics are determined by an interaction of genes on several chromosomes or at several places on one chromosome. This condition is polygenic inheritance. An example of polygenic inheritance is human skin colour.

Genes for skin colour are located in many places, and skin colour is determined by which genes are present at these multiple locations. A person with many genes for dark skin will have very dark skin colour, and a person with multiple genes for light skin will have very light skin colour. Many people have some genes for light skin and some for dark skin, which explains why so many variations of skin colour exist. Height is another characteristic probably reflecting polygenic characteristics.

PROTEIN BIOSYNTHESIS

Protein biosynthesis (synthesis) is the process in which cells build proteins. The term is sometimes used to refer only to protein translation but more often it refers to a multi-step process, beginning with amino acid synthesis and transcription which are then used for translation. Protein biosynthesis, although very similar, differs between prokaryotes and eukaryotes.

Amino acid synthesis

Amino acids are the monomers which are polymerized to produce proteins. Amino acid synthesis is the set of biochemical processes (metabolic pathways) which build the amino acids from carbon sources like glucose.

Not all amino acids may be synthesised by every organism, for example adult humans have to obtain 8 of the 20 amino acids from their diet.

Transcription

Transcription is the process by which an mRNA template, encoding the sequence of the protein in the form of a trinucleotide code, is transcribed from the genome to provide a template for translation. Transcription copies the template from one strand of the DNA double helix, called the template strand. Transcription can be divided into 3 stages: Initiation, Elongation and Termination, each regulated by a large number of proteins such as transcription factors and coactivators that ensure the correct gene is transcribed in response to appropriate signals. The DNA strand is read in the 3' to 5' direction and the mRNA is transcribed in the 5' to 3' direction by the RNA polymerase.

Translation

The synthesis of proteins is known as translation. Translation occurs in the cytoplasm where the ribosomes are located. Ribosomes are made of a small and large subunit which surrounds the mRNA.

In translation, messenger RNA (mRNA) is decoded to produce a specific polypeptide according to the rules specified by the genetic code. This uses an mRNA sequence as a template to guide the synthesis of a chain of amino acids that form a protein. Translation is necessarily preceded by transcription. Translation proceeds in four phases: activation, initiation, elongation and termination (all describing the growth of the amino acid chain, or polypeptide that is the product of translation). In activation, the correct amino acid (AA) is joined to the correct transfer RNA (tRNA). While this is not technically a step in translation, it is required for translation to proceed. The AA is joined by its carboxyl group to the 3' OH of the tRNA by an ester bond. When the tRNA has an amino acid linked to it, it is termed "charged". Initiation involves the small subunit of the ribosome binding to 5' end of mRNA with the help of initiation factors (IF), other proteins that assist the process.

Elongation occurs when the next aminoacyl-tRNA (charged tRNA) in line binds to the ribosome along with GTP and an elongation factor. Termination of the polypeptide happens when the A site of the ribosome faces a stop codon (UAA, UAG, or UGA). When this happens, no tRNA can recognize it, but releasing factor can recognize nonsense codons and causes the release of the polypeptide chain. The capacity of disabling or inhibiting translation in protein biosynthesis is used by antibiotics such as: anisomycin, cycloheximide, chloramphenicol, tetracycline, streptomycin, erythromycin, puromycin etc.

Events following protein translation

The events following biosynthesis include post-translational modification and protein folding. During and after synthesis, polypeptide chains often fold to assume, so called, native secondary and tertiary structures. This is known as *protein folding*. Many proteins undergo *post-translational modification*. This may include the formation of disulfide bridges or attachment of any of a number of biochemical functional groups, such as acetate, phosphate, various lipids and carbohydrates. Enzymes may also remove one or more amino acids from the leading (amino) end of the polypeptide chain, leaving a protein consisting of two polypeptide chains connected by disulfide bonds.

Peptide synthesis

In organic chemistry, peptide synthesis is the production of peptides, which are organic compounds in which multiple amino acids bind via peptide bonds which are also known as amide bonds. The biological process of producing long peptides (proteins) is known as protein biosynthesis.

Chemistry

Peptides are synthesized by coupling the carboxyl group or C-terminus of one amino acid to the amino group or N-terminus of another.

Liquid-phase Synthesis

Liquid-phase peptide synthesis is a classical approach to peptide synthesis. It has been replaced in most labs by solid-phase synthesis. However, it retains usefulness in large-scale production of peptides for industrial purposes.

Solid-phase Synthesis

Solid-phase peptide synthesis (SPPS), pioneered by Robert Bruce Merrifield, resulted in a paradigm shift within the peptide synthesis community. It is now the accepted method for creating peptides and proteins in the lab in a synthetic manner. SPPS allows the synthesis of natural peptides which are difficult to express in bacteria, the incorporation of unnatural amino acids, peptide/protein backbone modification, and the synthesis of D-proteins, which consist of D-amino acids.

Small solid beads, insoluble yet porous, are treated with functional units ('linkers') on which peptide chains can be built. The peptide will remain covalently attached to the bead until cleaved from it by a reagent such as trifluoroacetic acid. The peptide is thus 'immobilized' on the solid-phase and can be retained during a filtration process, whereas liquid-phase reagents and by-products of synthesis are flushed away.

The general principle of SPPS is one of repeated cycles of coupling-deprotection. The free N-terminal amine of a solid-phase attached peptide is coupled to a single N-protected amino acid unit. This unit is then deprotected, revealing a new N-terminal amine to which a further amino acid may be attached. The overwhelmingly important consideration is to generate extremely high yield in each step. For example, if each coupling step were to have 99% yield, a 26-amino acid peptide would be synthesized in 77% final yield (assuming 100% yield in each deprotection); if each step were 95%, it would be synthesized in 25% yield. Thus each amino acid is added in major excess (2~10x) and coupling amino acids together is highly optimized by a series of well-characterized agents.

There are two majorly used forms of SPPS — Fmoc and Boc. Unlike ribosome protein synthesis, solid-phase peptide synthesis proceeds in a C-terminal to N-terminal fashion. The N-termini of amino acid monomers is protected by these two groups and added onto a deprotected amino acid chain.

Automated synthesizers are available for both techniques, though many research groups continue to perform SPPS manually. SPPS is limited by yields, and typically peptides and proteins in the range of 70~100 amino acids are pushing the limits of synthetic accessibility. Synthetic difficulty also is sequence dependent; typically amyloid peptides and proteins are difficult to make. Longer lengths can be accessed by using native chemical ligation to couple two peptides together with quantitative yields.

t-Boc Solid-phase Peptide Synthesis

When Merrifield invented SPPS in 1963, it was according to the t-Boc method. t-Boc (or Boc) stands for (t)ert-(B)ut(o)xy(c)arbonyl. To remove Boc from a growing peptide chain, acidic conditions are used (usually neat TFA). Removal of side-chain protecting groups and the peptide from the resin at the end of the synthesis is achieved by incubating in hydrofluoric acid (which can be dangerous or even deadly); for this reason Boc chemistry is generally disfavored. Also, HF cleavage needs to be done in special fume hoods using specialized equipment. However for complex syntheses Boc is favourable. When synthesizing nonnatural peptide analogs which are base-sensitive (such as depsipeptides), Boc is necessary.

Fmoc Solid-phase Peptide Synthesis

This method was introduced by Carpino in 1972 and further applied by Atherton in 1978. Fmoc stands for 9*H*-(f)luoren-9-yl(m)eth(o)xy(c)arbonyl which describes the Fmoc protecting group, first described as a protecting group by Carpino in 1970. To remove an Fmoc from a growing peptide chain, basic conditions (usually 20% piperidine in DMF) are used. Removal of side-chain protecting groups and peptide from the resin is achieved by incubating in trifluoroacetic acid (TFA), deionized water, and triisopropylsilane. Fmoc deprotection is usually slow because the anionic nitrogen produced at the end is not a particularly favorable product, although the whole process is thermodynamically driven by the evolution of carbon dioxide. The main advantage of Fmoc chemistry is that no hydrofluoric acid is needed. It is therefore used for most routine synthesis.

Bop Spps

The use of BOP reagent was first described by Castro et al in 1975.

Solid supports

The physical properties of the solid support, and the applications to which it can be utilized, vary with the material from which the support is constructed, the amount of crosslinking, as well as the linker and handle being used.

Polystyrene Resin

Polystyrene resin is a versatile resin and it is quite useful in multi-well, automated peptide synthesis, due to its minimal swelling in dichloromethane.

Polyamide Resin

Polyamide resin is also a useful and versatile resin. It seems to swell much more than polystyrene, in which case it may not be suitable for some automated synthesizers, if the wells are too small.

PEG Based Resin

ChemMatrix(R) is a new type of resin which is based on PEG that is crosslinked. ChemMatrix(R) has claimed a high chemical and thermal stability (is compatible with Microwave synthesis) and has shown higher degrees of swellings in acetonitrile, dichloromethane, DMF, N-methyl pyrollidone, TFA and water compared to the polystyrene based resins. ChemMatrix has shown significant improvements to the synthesis of hydrophobic sequences. ChemMatrix is recommended for the synthesis of difficult and long peptides.

Protecting groups

Due to amino acid excesses used to ensure complete coupling during each synthesis step, polymerization of amino acids is common in reactions where each amino acid is not protected. In order to prevent this polymerization, protecting groups are used. This adds additional deprotection phases to the synthesis reaction, creating a repeating design flow as follows:

- Protective group is removed from trailing amino acids in a deprotection reaction
- Deprotection reagents washed away to provide clean coupling environment
- Protected amino acids dissolved in a solvent such as dimethylformamide (DMF) are combined with coupling reagents are pumped through the synthesis column
- Coupling reagents washed away to provide clean deprotection environment

Currently, two protective groups (t-Boc, Fmoc) are commonly used in solid-phase peptide synthesis. Their lability is caused by the carbamate group which readily releases CO_2 for an irreversible decoupling step.

t-Boc Protective Group

The t-Boc group was commonly used for protecting the terminal amine of the peptide, requiring the use of more acid stable groups for side chain protection in orthogonal strategies. It retains usefulness in reducing aggregation of peptides during synthesis. Boc groups can be added to amino acids with t-Boc anhydride and a suitable base.

Fmoc Pprotective Group

Fmoc (9H-fluoren-9-ylmethoxycarbonyl) is currently a widely used protective group that is generally removed from the N terminus of a peptide in the iterative synthesis of a peptide from amino acid units. The advantage of Fmoc is that it is cleaved under very mild basic conditions (e.g. piperidine), but stable under acidic conditions. This allows mild acid labile protecting groups that are stable under basic conditions, such as Boc and benzyl groups, to be used on the side-chains of amino acid residues of the target peptide. This orthogonal protecting group strategy is common in the art of organic synthesis. FMOC is preferred over BOC due to ease of cleavage; however it is less atom-economical, as the fluorenyl group is much larger than the tert-butyl group. Accordingly, prices for FMOC amino acids were high until the large-scale piloting of one of the first synthesized peptide drugs, enfuvirtide, began in the 1990s, when market demand adjusted the relative prices of the two sets of amino acids.

Benzyloxy-carbonyl (Z) Group

The first use of (Z) group as protecting groups was done by Max Bergmann who synthesised oligopeptides. Another carbamate based group is the benzyloxy-carbonyl (Z) group. It is removed in harsher conditions: HBr/acetic acid or catalytic hydrogenation. Today it is almost exclusively used for side chain protection.

Alloc Protecting Group

The allyloxycarbonyl (alloc) protecting group is often used to protect a carboxylic acid, hydroxyl, or amino group when an orthogonal deprotection scheme is required. It is sometimes used when conducting on-resin cyclic peptide formation, where the peptide is linked to the resin by a side-chain functional group. The alloc group can be removed using tetrakis (triphenylphosphine)palladium(0) along with a 37:2:1 mixture of chloroform, acetic acid, and N-methylmorpholine (NMM) for 2 hours. The resin must then be carefully washed 0.5% DIPEA in DMF, 3x10 ml of 0.5% sodium diethylthiocarbamate in DMF, and then 5x10 ml of 1:1 DCM:DMF.

Lithographic Protecting Groups

For special applications like protein microarrays lithographic protecting groups are used. Those groups can be removed through exposure to light.

Activating groups

For coupling the peptides the carboxyl group is usually activated. This is important for speeding up the reaction. There are two main types of activating groups: carbodiimides and triazolols.

Carbodiimides

These activating agents were first developed. Most common are dicyclohexylcarbodiimide (DCC) and diisopropylcarbodiimide (DIC). Reaction with a carboxylic acid yields a highly reactive O-acyl-urea. During artificial protein synthesis (such as Fmoc solid-state synthesizers), the C-terminus is often used as the attachment site on which the amino acid monomers are added. To enhance the electrophilicity of carboxylate group, the negatively charged oxygen must first be "activated" into a better leaving group. DCC is used for this purpose. The negatively charged oxygen will act as a nucleophile, attacking the central carbon in DCC. DCC is temporarily attached to the former carboxylate group (which is now an ester group), making nucleophilic attack by an amino group (on the attaching amino acid) to the former C-terminus (carbonyl group) more efficient. The problem with carbodiimides is that they are too reactive and that they can therefore cause racemization of the amino acid.

Triazolols

To solve the problem of racemization, triazolols were introduced. The most important ones are 1-hydroxy-benzotriazole (HOBt) and 1-hydroxy-7-aza-benzotriazole (HOAt). Others have been developed. These substances can react with the O-acylurea to form an active ester which is less reactive and less in danger of racemization. HOAt is especially favourable because of a neighbouring group effect.

Newer developments omit the carbodiimides totally. The active ester is introduced as a uronium or phosphonium salt of a non-nucleophilic anion (tetrafluoroborate or hexafluorophosphate): HBTU, HATU, PyBOP.

Synthesizing long peptides

Stepwise elongation, in which the amino acids are connected step-by-step in turn, is ideal for small peptides containing between 2 and 100 amino acid residues. Another method is fragment condensation, in which peptide fragments are coupled. Although the former can elongate the peptide chain without racemization, the yield drops if only it is used in the creation of long or highly polar peptides. Fragment condensation is better than stepwise elongation for synthesizing sophisticated long peptides, but its use must be restricted in order to protect against racemization. Fragment condensation is also undesirable since the coupled fragment must be in gross excess, which may be a limitation depending on the length of the fragment.

A new development for producing longer peptide chains is chemical ligation: Unprotected peptide chains react chemoselectively in aqueous solution. A first kinetically controlled product rearranges to form the amide bond. The most common form of native chemical ligation uses a peptide thioester that reacts with a terminal cystein residue.

MICROWAVE ASSISTED PEPTIDE SYNTHESIS

Although microwave irradiation has been around since the late 1940s, it was not until 1986 that microwave energy was used in organic chemistry. During the end of the 1980s and 1990s, microwave energy was an obvious source for completing chemical reactions in minutes that would otherwise take several hours to days. Through several technical improvements at the end of the 1990s and beginning of the 2000s, microwave synthesizers have been designed to provide both low and high energy pockets of microwave energy so that the temperature of the reaction mixture could controlled. The microwave energy used in peptide synthesis is of a single frequency providing maximum penetration depth of the sample which is in contrast to conventional kitchen microwaves. In peptide synthesis, microwave irradiation has been used to complete long peptide sequences with high degrees of yield and low degrees of racemization. Microwave irradiation during the coupling of amino acids to a growing polypeptide chain is not only catalyzed through the increase in temperature, but also due to the alternating electromagnetic radiation to which the polar backbone of the polypeptide continuously aligns to.

Due to the this phenomenon, the microwave energy can prevent aggregation and thus increases yields of the final peptide product. Despite the main advantages of microwave irradiation of peptide synthesis, the main disadvantage is the racemization which may occur with the coupling of cysteine and histidine. A typical coupling reaction with these amino acids are performed at lower temperatures than the other 18 natural amino acids. Another disadvantage is that allyl containing amino acid derivatives cannot be coupled to amino acids using microwave irradiation due to uncontrolled polymerization.

3

Basics of Structure and Analysis of DNA

CENTRAL DOGMA

The following diagram displays the flow of genetic information from DNA to the protein. This can be interpreted in genetic terms by saying that information contained in genes (DNA) is eventually expressed as the phenotype (protein).

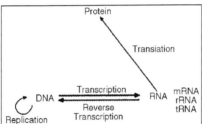

Compartmentalisation of the Central Dogma of Molecular Genetics

The organelles of plants are both of a prokaryotic (chloroplast and mitochondria) and eukaryotic (nucleaus) origin. The organelles contain DNA as well as the nucleus. Also, found within each organelle are all of the steps of the central dogma of molecular genetics. Reverse transcription has not been demonstrated in the organelles, but plant mitochondria undergo mRNA editing, a feature not known for nuclear expressed genes.

Definition of Gene

Many molecular definitions of a gene relate to their role in directing the production of specific proteins. This stems from the analysis of mutants where it was shown that the absence of a specific protein was related to the mutation. Proteins are key components in the central dogma as polymerases but they also have other key metabolic roles.

These role are:

• Enzymatic
• Structural components
• Regulatory roles

Original Concept of the Gene: One gene = one Enzyme

This concept does not hold for those proteins that are heteromeric or consist two of two or more different subunits.

Example: RUBISCO (ribulose bisphosphate carboxylase oxygenase)

$$CO_2 + \text{5-C-sugar} \rightarrow 2 \text{ 3-C-sugars}$$

RUBISCO is a multimeric protein of 16 peptides:

• 8 small subunits (nuclear encoded)
• 8 large subunits (chloroplast encoded)
  – Thus two genes are responsible for this enzyme

Revised Concept: One gene = one peptide

Newest Discovery

Glucose 6-phosphate dehydrogenase is an enzyme found in human red blood cells.

The major form this peptide is encoded from information from two chromosomes.

• *Minor form*: NH_4 — — — — —CO_3

(The sequences encoding the gene are on the X chromosome.)

• *Major form*: NH_4xx— — — — —CO_3

(Amino acids 1-53 are encoded on chromosome 6, and amino acids 54-479 are encoded on the X chromosome.)

• *Conclusion*: This gene fits the one gene = one peptide model stated above, if you are willing to accept that not all genes reside on a single continuous stretch of DNA.

Proof that DNA is Genetic Material

Griffith

When he added dead, virulent pneumonia bacteria to a mouse, it lived; but if he added dead virulent bacteria to live non-virulent bacteria some mice died.

He termed the material that changed the non-virulent bacteria to virulent thetransforming principle.

Avery, MacLeod and McCarty

They used biochemical purification of cellular fractions to determine that DNA and not RNA or protein was the transforming principle. Transformation - the alteration of phenotype by the addition of foreign DNA

Hershey and Chase The "Blender Experiment"

They knew that:

DNA - has P but no S

Protein - has S but not P

They also knew that something from T2 phage entered *E. coli* cells and directed the bacteria to produce more phage. They assumed that the genetic material was the material that entered the cell. So they set out to determine the chemical nature of the material. In separate experiments they infected *E. coli* cells with 35S or 32P labeled phage. By analyzing the products they determined that 32P entered the cell. Thus DNA must be the genetic material.

DRUG ACTING ON DNA

Mechanism of Intercalating

Intercalating agents wedge between bases along the DNA. The intercalated drug molecules affect the structure of the DNA, preventing polymerases and other DNA binding proteins from functioning properly. The result is prevention of DNA synthesis, inhibition of transcription and induction of mutations. The effect of principal alkaloids (sanguinarine, chelerythrine, coptisine, chelidonine) of greater celandine Chelidonium majus L., as well as the alkaloids from Colchicum autumnale L.(colchicine and colchamine) on calcium accumulation and oxidative phosphorylation in rat liver mitochondria has been studied. The obtained data were compared with DNA intercalating properties of alkaloids detected by the method of thermodenaturation (DNA melting curve plots). It was found that chelerythrine and sanguinarine blocked absorption and accumulation of calcium cations and inhibited oxidative phosphorylation, while the coptisine significantly diminished those indices. Chelidonine, colchicines and colchamine had no influence on the studied characteristics. The effect of alkaloids upon mitochondria functional state correlated tightly with their DNA intercalating properties: chelerythrine and sanguinarine were strong intercalators, while coptisine was a weak one, and chelidonine, colchicine and colchamine did not interact with DNA and caused no changes in its melting point.

Correlation coefficient between the intercalating properties of alkaloids and their inhibition of calcium accumulation was 0.89, and with their oxidative phosphorylation inhibition -0.93. It is suggested that the effect of studied alkaloids upon functional properties of mitochondria can be mediated by mtDNA. DNA topoisomerase I is essential for cellular metabolism and survival. It is also the target of a novel class of anticancer drugs active against previously refractory solid tumors, the camptothecins.

The present review describes the topoisomerase I catalytic mechanisms with particular emphasis on the cleavage complex that represents the enzyme's catalytic intermediate and the site of action for camptothecins. Roles of topoisomerase I in DNA replication, transcription and recombination are also reviewed. Because of the importance of topoisomerase I as a chemotherapeutic target, we review the mechanisms of action of camptothecins and the other topoisomerase I inhibitors identified to date.

The DNA intercalating agents 4'-(9-acridinyl-amino) methanesulfon-m-anisidide (m-AMSA) and adriamycin were studied by using filter elution methods to measure DNA single-strand breaks (SSB's), DNA-protein cross-links (DPC's), and double-stranded breaks (DSB's) in mouse leukemia L1210 cells. Both compounds produced SSB's and DPC's at nearly 1:1 ratios. The SSB's and DPC's were shown to be localised with respect to each other; this was inferred from the finding that filter assays based on protein adsorption completely prevented the elution of the DNA single-strand segments between SSB's. In the case of m-AMSA, which produces relatively high frequencies of DNA lesions, the possibility that a protein bridges across the SSB was excluded by alkaline sedimentation studies.

The o-AMSA isomer is much less cytotoxic than m-AMSA and did not produce protein-associated strand breaks. The simplest model to explain the results is that a protein becomes covalently bound to either the 3' or the 5' termini of the intercalator-induced strand breaks. At moderately cytotoxic doses, m-AMSA yielded much larger frequencies of protein-associated SSB's than did adriamycin. m-AMSA-induced protein-associated SSB's saturated at approximately 60000 per cell over a concentration range in which m-AMSA uptake by the cells was proportional to the drug concentration. m-AMSA was found to enter and exit from cells very rapidly at 37 degrees C; protein-associated SSB's and DSB's also appeared and disappeared rapidly. At reduced temperature, however, the appearance and disappearance of protein-associated SSB's could be blocked while m-AMSA entry and exit still occurred.

The saturation behaviour and temperature dependence suggest that the formation and disappearance of protein-associated strand breaks is enzymatic. The simplest hypothesis is that the linked protein is a nuclease, such as a topoisomerase, which becomes bound to one terminus of the strand break it produces. It is proposed that topoisomerases producing SSB's and DSB's are stimulated to different degrees by different intercalators. Topoisomerase II mediated DNA scission induced by both a non-intercalating agent [4'-demethylepipodophyllotoxin 4-(4,6-O-ethylidene-beta-D glucopyrano-side)(VP-16)] and an intercalator [4'-(9-acridinylamino) methanesulfon-m-anisidide (m-AMSA)] wasstudied as a function of proliferation in Chinese hamster ovary (CHO), HeLa, and mouse leukemia L1210 cell lines. Log-phase CHO cells exhibited dose-dependent drug-induced DNA breaks, while plateau cells were found to be resistant to the effects of VP-16 and m-AMSA. Neither decreased viability nor altered drug uptake accounted for the drug resistance of these confluent cells. In contrast to CHO cells, plateau-phase HeLa and L1210 cells remained sensitive to VP-16 and m-AMSA. Recovery of drug sensitivity by plateau-phase CHO cells was found to reach a maximum approximately 18 h after these cells regained exponential growth and was independent of DNA synthesis.

DNA strand break frequency correlated with cytotoxicity in CHO cells; log cells demonstrated an inverse log linear relationship between drug dose (or DNA damage) and colony survival, whereas plateau-derived colony survival was virtually unaffected by increasing drug dose. Topoisomerase II activity, whether determined by decatenation of kinetoplast DNA, by cleavage of pBR322 DNA, or by precipitation of the DNA-topoisomerase II complex, was uniformly severalfold greater in log-phase CHO cells compared to plateau-phase cells.

The biochemical characteristics of the formation and disappearance of intercalator-induced DNA double-strand breaks (DSB) were studied in nuclei from mouse leukemia L1210 cells by using filter elution methodology. The three intercalators used were 4'-(9-acridinylamino)-methanesulfon-m-anisidide (m-AMSA), 5-iminodaunorubicin (5-ID), and ellipticine. These compounds differ in that they produced predominantly DNA single-strand breaks (SSB)(m-AMSA) or predominantly DNA double-strand breaks (ellipticine) or a mixture of both SSB and DSB (5-ID) in whole cells. In isolated nuclei, each intercalator produced DSB at a frequency comparable to that which is produced in whole cells. Moreover, these DNA breaks reversed within 30 min after drug removal. It thus appeared that neither ATP nor other nucleotides were necessary for intercalator-dependent DNA nicking-closing reactions. The formation of the intercalator-induced DSB was reduced at ice temperature. Break formation was also reduced in the absence of magnesium, at a pH above 6.4 and at NaCl concentrations above 200 mM. In the presence of ATP and ATP analogues, the intercalator-induced cleavage was enhanced. These results suggest that the intercalator-induced DSB are enzymatically mediated and that the enzymes involved in these reactions can catalyse DNA double-strand cleavage and rejoining in the absence of ATP, although the occupancy of an ATP binding site might convert the enzyme to a form more reactive to intercalators. Three inhibitors of DNA topoisomerase II—novobiocin, nalidixic acid, and norfloxacin—reduced the formation of DNA strand breaks.

Mechanisms of Alkylating Agents

Alkylating agents work by three different mechanisms all of which achieve the same end result - disruption of DNA function and cell death.In the first mechanism an alkylating agent (represented in the figure below as a pink star) attaches alkyl groups (small carbon compounds-depicted as pink triangles) to DNA bases. This alteration results in the DNA being fragmented by repair enzymes in their attempts to replace the alkylated bases (frame 3 of the diagram below). Alkylated bases prevent DNA synthesis and RN transcription from the affected DNA.

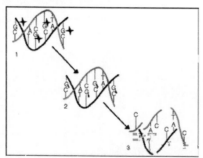

A second mechanism by which alkylating agents cause DNA damage is the formation of cross-bridges, bonds between atoms in the DNA. In this process, two bases are linked together by an alkylating agent that has two DNA binding sites. Bridges can be formed within a single molecule of DNA (as shown below) or a cross-bridge may connect two different DNA molecules. Cross-linking prevents DNA from being separated for synthesis or transcription.

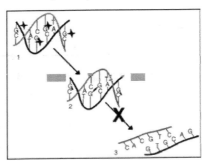

The third mechanism of action of alkylating agents is the induction of mispairing of the nucleotidesleading to mutations. In a normal DNA double helix, A always pairs with (is across from) T and G always pairs with C. As the figure below shows, alkylated G bases may erroneously pair with Ts. If this altered pairing is not corrected it may lead to a permanent mutation. Alkylating agents are one of the earliest and most commonly used chemotherapy agents used for cancer treatments. Their use in cancer treatments started in early 1940s. Majority of alkaline agents are active or dormant nitrogen mustards, which are poisonous compound initially used for certain military purposes. Chlorambucil, Cyclophosphamide, CCNU, Melphalan, Procarbazine, Thiotepa, BCNU, and Busulfan are some of the commonly used alkylating agents.

Although they might differ in their clinical activity, action mechanism of all alkylating agents is the same. These agents work directly on the DNA and prevent the cell division process by cross-linking and breaking the DNA strands and causing abnormal base pairing. When a DNA is altered in this manner, undesired cellular activity comes to a halt and the cell dies eventually.

Alkylating chemotherapy drugs are effective during all phases of cell cycle. Therefore, they are used to treat a large number of cancers. However, they are more effective in treating slow-growing cancers such as solid tumors and leukemia. Long term use of alkylating agents can lead to permanent infertility by decreasing sperm production in males, and causing menstruation cessation in females. Many alkylating agents can also lead to secondary cancers such as Acute Myeloid Leukemia, years after the therapy.

Antimetabolites

Structure of antimetabolites (antineoplastic agents) is similar to certain compounds such as vitamins, amino acids, and precursors of DNA or RNA, found naturally in human body. Antimetabolites help in treatment cancer by inhibiting cell division thereby hindering the growth of tumor cells. These agents get incorporated in the DNA or RNA to interfere with the process of division of cancer cells. Antimetabolites were first discovered and it is found that folic acid analog can reduce childhood leukemia. Out of 16 patients he tested, 10 displayed hematologic improvement. This discovery laid the foundation that enabled scientist to synthesise many new agents that could inhibit biological enzymatic reactions. Antimetabolites are found to be useful in treating chronic and acute cases of leukemia and various tumors. They are commonly used to treat gastrointestinal tract, breast, and ovary tumors.

Methotraxate, which is a commonly used antimetabolites chemotherapy agent, is effective in the S-phase of the cell cycle. It works by inhibiting an enzyme that is essential for DNA synthesis. 6-mercaptopurine and 5-fluorouracil (5FU) are two other commonly used antimetabolites. 5-Fluorouracil (5-FU) works by interfering with the DNA components, nucleotide, to stop DNA synthesis. This drug is used to treat many different types of cancers including breast, esophageal, head, neck, and gastric cancers. 6-mercaptopurine is an analogue of hypoxanthine and is commonly used to treat Acute Lymphoblastic Leukemia (ALL). Other popular antimetabolite chemotherapy drugs are Thioguanine, Cytarabine, Cladribine. Gemcitabine, and Fludarabine.

Anthracyclines

Anthracyclines were developed between 1970s and 1990s and are daunosamine and tetra-hydronaphthacenedione-based chemotherapy agents. These compounds are cell-cycle non-specific and are used to treat a large number of cancers including lymphomas, leukemia, and uterine, ovarian, lung and breast cancers.

Anthracyclines drugs are developed from natural resources. For instance, daunorubicin is developed by isolating it from soil-dwelling fungus Streptomyces. Similarly, Doxorubicin, which is another commonly used anthracycline chemotherapy agent, is isolated from mutated strain of Streptomyces. Although both the drugs have similar clinical action mechanisms, doxorubicin is more effective in treating solid tumors. Idarubicin, Epirubicin, and Mitoxantrone are few of the other commonly used anthracycline chemotherapy drugs. Anthracyclines work by forming free oxygen radicals that breaks DNA strands thereby inhibiting DNA synthesis and function. These chemotherapeutic agents form a complex with DNA and enzyme to inhibit the topoisomerase enzyme. Topoisomerase is an enzyme class that causes the supercoiling of DNA, allowing DNA repair, transcription, and replication.

One of the main side effects of anthracyclines is that it can damage cells of heart muscle along with the DNA of cancer cell leading to cardiac toxicity.

Antitumor Antibiotics

Antitumor antibiotics are also developed from the soil fungus Streptomyces. These drugs are widely used to treat and suppress development of tumors in the body. Similar to anthracyclines, antitumor antibiotics drugs also form free oxygen radicals that result in DNA strand breaks, killing the growth of cancer cells. In most of the cases, these drugs are used in combination with other chemotherapy agents. Bleomycin is one of the commonly used antitumor antibiotic used to treat testicular cancer and hodgkin's lymphoma. The most serious side effect of this drug is lung toxicity that occurs when the oxygen radical formed by the antitumor antibiotics damages lung cells along with the cancer cells.

Monoclonal Antibodie

Monoclonal antibodies are one of the newer chemotherapy agents approved for cancer treatment by the Food and Drug Administration (FDA) in 1997. Alemtuzumab (Campath), Bevacizumab (Avastin), Cetuximab (Erbitux), Gemtuzumab (Mylotarg), Ibritumomab (Zevalin), Panitumumab (Vectibix), Rituximab (Rituxan), Tositumomab (Bexxar), and Trastuzumab (Herceptin) are some of the FDA approved monoclonal drugs used in chemotherapeutic cancer treatments. The treatment is known to be useful in treating colon, lung, head, neck, and breast cancers.

Some of the monoclonal drugs are used to treat chronic lymphocytic leukemia, acute myelogenous leukemia, and non-Hodgkin's lymphoma. Monoclonal antibodies work by attaching to certain parts of the tumor-specific antigens and make them easily recognisable by the host's immune system. They also prevent growth of cancer cells by blocking the cell receptors to which chemicals called 'growth factors' attach promoting cell growth. Monoclonal antibodies can be combined with radioactive particles and other powerful anticancer drugs to deliver them directly to cancer cells. Using this method, long term radioactive treatment and anticancer drugs can be given to patients without causing any serious harm to other healthy cells of the body.

Platinums

Platinum-based natural metal derivatives were found to be useful for cancer treatments around 150 years ago with the synthesis of cisplatin.

However, there clinical use did not commence until 30 years ago. Platinum-based chemotherapy agents work by cross-linking subunits of DNA. These agents act during any part of cell cycle and help in treating cancer by impairing DNA synthesis, transcription, and function.

Cisplatin, although found to be useful in treating testicular and lung cancer, is highly toxic and can severely damage the kidneys of the patient. Second generation platinum-complex carboplatin is found to be much less toxic in comparison to cisplatin and has fewer kidney-related side effects.

Oxaliplatin, which is third generation platinum-based complex, is found to be helpful in treating colon cancer. Although, oxaliplatin does not cause any toxicity in kidney it can lead to severe neuropathies.

Plant Alkaloids

Plant alkaloid chemotherapy agents, as the name suggests, are plant derivatives. They are cell-specific chemotherapy agents. However, the cycle affected is based on the drug used for the treatment. They are primarily categorised into four groups: topoisomerase inhibitors, vinca alkaloids, taxanes, and epipodophyllotoxins. Plant alkaloids are cell-cycle specific, but the cycle affected varies from drug to drug. Vincristine (Oncovin) is a plant alkaloid of interest in mesothelioma treatment.

Topoisomerase Inhibitors

Topoisomerase inhibitors are chemotherapy agents are categorised into Type I and Type II Topoisomerases inhibitors and they work by interfering with DNA transcription, replication, and function to prevent DNA supercoiling.

- *Type I Topoisomerase inhibitors:* These chemotherapy agents are extracted from the bark and wood of the Chinese tree Camptotheca accuminata. They work by forming a complex with topoisomerase DNA. This in turn suppresses the function of topoisomerase.

  Camptothecins which includes irinotecan and topotecan are commonly used type I topoisomerase inhibitors, first discovered in the late 1950s.

- *Type II Topoisomerase inhibitors:* These are extracted from the alkaloids found in the roots of May Apple plants. They work in the in the work in the late S and G2 phases of the cell cycle.

  Amsacrine, etoposide, etoposide phosphate, and teniposide are some of the examples of type II topoisomerase inhibitors.

Vinca Alkaloids

Vinca alkaloids are derived from the periwinkle plant, Vinca rosea (Catharanthus roseus) and are known to be used by the natives of Madagascar to treat diabetes. Although not useful in controlling diabetes, vinca alkaloids, are useful in treating leukemias. They are effective in the M phase of the cell cycle and work by inhibiting tubulin assembly in microtubules. Vincristine, Vinblastine, Vinorelbine, and Vindesine are some of the popularly used vinca alkaloid chemotherapy agents used today. Major side effect of vinca alkaloids is that they can cause neurotoxicity in patients.

Taxanes

Taxanes are plant alkaloids that were first developed in 1963 by isolating it from first isolated from the bark of the Pacific yew tree, Taxus brevifolia in 1963. Paclitaxel, which is the active components of taxanes was first discovered in 1971 and was made available for clinical use in the year 1993. Taxanes also work in the M-phase of the cell cycle and inhibit the function of microtubules by binding with them. Paclitaxel and docetaxel are commonly used taxanes. Taxanes chemotherapy agents are used to treat a large array of cancers including breast, ovarian, lung, head and neck, gastric, esophageal, prostrate and gastric cancers. The main side effect of taxanes is that they lower the blood counts in patients.

DNA STRUCTURE

Watson and Crick Model of DNA

The following are the features of the DNA molecule as described by Watson and Crick in 1953:

- 2 chains
- purine opposite a pyrimidine
- chains held together by H-bonds
  - Guanine is paired with cytosine by three H-bonds
  - Adenine is paired with thymine by two H-bonds
- Anti-parallel orientation of the two chains

  $5' \rightarrow 3'$

  $3' \leftarrow 5'$
- The molecule is stabilised by:
  - Large # of H-bonds
  - Hydrophobic bonding between the stacked bases

Components of DNA

DNA is composed of two chains of repeating nucleotides. Each nucleotide consists of three components.

These components are:

- Phosphate Group
- 2-deoxyribose sugar
- A nitrogen containing base
    - Cytosine
    - Adenine
    - Guanine
    - Thymine

Types of DNA

The DNA molecule that Watson and Crick described was in the B form. It is now known that DNA can exist in several other forms. The primary difference between the forms is the direction that the helix spirals.

A, B, C = right-handed helix

Z = left-handed helix (found *in vitro* under high salt)

B is the major form that is found in the cell. Z-DNA was initially found only under high salt conditions, but the cellular environment is actually a low-salt environment. The question then is whether type Z exist under cellular conditions. Several features have been discovered that can stablise Z-DNA under in a low salt environment.

- Alternating purine/pyrimidine tracts
    - Poly GC or poly AT stretches
- 5-methyl-cytosine

Because both of these conditions can exists in the cell, it is suggested that stretches of Z-DNA may actually exists in the cell along with other stretches of B-DNA. In addition to the direction the molecule turns, several other differences exists between the various forms of DNA. The following table summarises the features of the different forms of DNA.

Form	Direction	Bases/360° Turn	Helix Diametre
A	Right	11.0	23A
B	Right	10.0	19A
C	Right	9.3	19A
Z	Left	12.0	18A

THE STRUCTURE OF DNA

The structure of DNA encodes all the information every cell needs to function and thrive. In addition, DNA carries hereditary information in a form that can be copied and passed intact from generation to generation.

```
┌─────────────────────────────────────────┐
│ Reading Frames                           │
│                                          │
│   A A A  C C U  A A G  G C C             │
│                                          │
│    Lys     Pro    Lys     Ala            │
│                                          │
│   A  A A C  C U A  A G G  C C            │
│                                          │
│      Asa     Lov     Arg   (Pro)         │
│                                          │
│   A A  A C C  U A A  G G C  C            │
│                                          │
│        Thr      STOP  (untranslatod)     │
└─────────────────────────────────────────┘
```

Fig. Genetic Code

A gene is a segment of DNA. The biochemical instructions found within most genes, known as the genetic code, specify the chemical structure of a particular protein. Proteins are composed of long chains of amino acids, and the specific sequence of these amino acids dictates the function of each protein. The DNA structure of a gene determines the arrangement of amino acids in a protein, ultimately determining the type and function of the protein manufactured.

Protein Synthesis

DNA replication ensures that the genetic instructions encoded in DNA can be used continuously through generations to produce the proteins that build and operate the cells of an organism. The process of tapping the genetic code to create proteins, known as protein synthesis, has two crucial steps: transcription and translation.

DNA Replication

In order for inherited traits to be transmitted from parent to child, the genetic information encoded in DNA must be copied with great precision during cell division. The accuracy of DNA replication depends upon the complementary pairing of bases. During replication, the DNA double helix unwinds and bonds joining the base pairs break, separating the DNA molecule into two separate strands. Each strand of DNA directs the synthesis of another complementary strand. The unpaired bases of each DNA strand attach to bases floating within the cell. But the DNA strand's unpaired bases bond only with specific, complementary bases—for example, an adenine base will bond only with a thymine base and a cytosine bases will pair only with a guanine base. Once all of the bases of a DNA strand bond to complementary bases, the complementary bases then link to each other, forming a new DNA double-helix molecule. Thus the original DNA molecule replicates into two DNA molecules that are exact duplicates.

Transcription

Transcription transfers the genetic code from a molecule of DNA to an intermediary molecule called ribonucleic acid (RNA). The basic nucleotide structure of RNA resembles that of DNA, but the two compounds have three critical differences. First, the structure of RNA incorporates the sugar ribose rather than deoxyribose, the sugar in DNA. Second, RNA uses the base uracil (U) instead of thymine (T). In RNA uracil binds with adenine just as thymine does in DNA. Third, RNA usually exists as a single strand, unlike the double-helix structure that normally characterizes DNA. Transcription involves the production of a special kind of RNA known as messenger RNA (mRNA).

The process begins when the two strands of a DNA molecule separate, a task directed by the enzyme RNA polymerase. After the double helix splits apart, one of the strands serves as a template, or pattern, for the formation of a complementary mRNA molecule. Free-floating individual bases within the cell bind to the bases on the DNA template using complementary base pairing. The individual bases then link together to form a strand of mRNA.

In eukaryotes (organisms whose cells have a nucleus), the mRNA strand undergoes an additional step before the next stage of protein synthesis can occur. The mRNA strand consists of coding regions called exons separated by regions called introns. The introns do not contribute to protein synthesis. Special enzymes in the nucleus remove the introns from the mRNA strand. The remaining exons then link together to form an mRNA strand that contains the entire code for making a protein.

Translation

Once transcription is complete and the genetic code has been copied onto mRNA, the genetic code must be converted into the language of proteins. That is, the information coded in the four bases found in mRNA must be translated into the instructions encoded by the 20 amino acids used in the formation of proteins. This process, called translation, takes place in cellular organelles called ribosomes.

In eukaryotes, mRNA travels out of the nucleus into the cell body to attach to a ribosome. In prokaryotes (organisms without a nucleus), the ribosome clasps mRNA and starts translation before these strands have finished transcription and separated from the DNA. In both eukaryotes and prokaryotes, the ribosome acts like a workbench and clamp that holds the mRNA strand and coordinates the activity of enzymes and other molecules essential to translation.

Another form of RNA called transfer RNA (tRNA) is found in the cytoplasm of the cell. There are many different types of tRNA, and each type binds with one of the 20 amino acids used in protein formation. One end of a tRNA binds with a specific amino acid. The other end carries three bases, known as an anticodon. The tRNA with an amino acid attached travels to the ribosome where the mRNA is stationed.

The anticodon of the tRNA undergoes complementary base pairing with a series of three bases on the mRNA, known as the codon. The mRNA codon codes for the type of amino acid carried by the tRNA. A second tRNA bonds with the next codon on the mRNA. The resident tRNA transfers its amino acid to the amino acid of the incoming tRNA and then leaves the ribosome.

This process continues repeatedly, with new tRNA receiving the growing chain of amino acids, known as a polypeptide chain, from a resident tRNA. The ribosome moves the mRNA strand one codon at a time, making new codons available to bind with tRNAs. The process ends when the entire sequence of mRNA has been translated. The polypeptide chain falls away from the ribosome as a newly formed protein, ready to go to work in the cell.

Mutations

Occasionally mistakes occur during DNA replication and protein synthesis. Any alteration in the structure of a gene results in a mutation. Mutations occur during DNA replication when the chemical structure of genes undergoes random modifications. Once a change has occurred, the altered genes continue to replicate in their changed form unless another mutation occurs. Sometimes mutations occur during transcription or translation, causing protein synthesis to go awry. Although mutations may occur in any living cell, they are most important when they occur in gametes because then the change affects the traits of following generations. Most mutations harm an organism. If a mutation occurs in a gene sequence that codes for a particular protein, the mutation may result in a change in the amino acid sequence directed by the gene. This change, in turn, may affect the function of the protein. The implications can be significant: The amino acid sequence distinguishing normal hemoglobin from the altered form of hemoglobin responsible for sickle-cell anemia differs by only a single amino acid. Some mutations may be neutral or silent and do not affect the function of a protein. Occasionally a mutation benefits an organism. Over the course of evolutionary time, however, mutations serve the crucial role of providing organisms with previously nonexistent proteins.

In this way, mutations are a driving force behind genetic diversity and the rise of new or more competitive species better able to adapt to changes, such as climate variations, depletion of food sources, or the emergence of new types of disease.

Mutations can produce a change in any region of a DNA molecule. In a *point mutation*, for example, a single nucleotide replaces another nucleotide. Although a point mutation produces a small change to the DNA sequence, it may cause a change in the amino acid sequence, and thus the function, of a protein. Far more serious are mutations that involve the addition or deletion of one or more bases from a DNA molecule.

Adding or subtracting even a single base from a normal sequence during transcription can disrupt translation by shifting the "reading frame" of every subsequent codon. For example, an mRNA strand may include two codons in the following sequence: AUG UGA. The addition of a cytosine base at the beginning of this sequence shifts the "spelling" of these codons so that they read: CAU GUG.

This may result in an incorrect amino acid sequence during translation, or the protein may be truncated. Known as frameshift mutation, this type of alteration could result in the production of a protein with no real function or one with a harmful effect.

Sometimes mutations are caused by transposition, in which long stretches of DNA (containing one or more genes) move from one chromosome to another. These jumping genes, called transposons, can disrupt transcription and change the type of amino acids inserted into a protein. Transposons rearrange and interrupt genes in a way that generally improves the genetic variation of a species.

While mutations can occur spontaneously, some can be caused by exposure to physical or chemical agents in the environment called mutagens.

Common environmental mutagens include ultraviolet rays from the sun and various chemicals, such as asbestos, cigarette smoke, and nitrous acid.

High-energy radiation, such as medical X rays, can cause DNA strands to break, leading to the deletion of potentially important genetic information. Radiation damage can also affect an entire chromosome, disrupting the function of many genes. In chromosomal translocation, a piece of one chromosome breaks off and merges with another chromosome. In some cases, large sections of chromosomes may break off and be lost. The cell has highly effective self-repair mechanisms that can correct the harmful changes made by mutations and prevent some mutations from being passed on. Some 50 specialized enzymes locate different types of faulty sequences in the DNA and clip out those flaws. Another repair mechanism scans DNA after replication and marks mismatched base pairs for repair.

GENES IN DEVELOPMENT

Gene regulation helps individual cells within an organism function in a specialized way. Other regulatory mechanisms coordinate the genes that determine how cells develop. All of the specialized cells in an organism, including those of the skin, muscle, bone, liver, and brain, derive from identical copies of a single fertilized egg cell. Each of these cells has the exact same DNA as the original cell, even though they have vastly different appearances and functions. Genes dictate how these cells specialize.

Early in an organism's embryonic development the overall body plan forms. Individual cells commit to a particular layer and region of the embryo, often migrating from one location to another to do so. As the organism grows, cells become part of a particular body organ or tissue, such as skin or muscle. Ultimately, most cells become highly specialized—not only to develop into a neuron rather than a muscle cell, for example, but to become a sensory neuron instead of a motor neuron.

This process of specialization is called differentiation. At each stage of the differentiation process, specific genes known as developmental control genes actively turn on and switch off the genes that differentiate cells. One class of developmental control genes, known as homeotic genes, directs the formation of particular body parts. Activating one set of homeotic genes instructs part of an embryo to develop into a leg, for example, while another set initiates the formation of the head.

If a homeotic gene becomes altered or damaged, an organism's body development can be dramatically disrupted. A change in a single gene in some insects, for instance, can cause a leg to grow where an antenna belongs. Homeotic genes work by regulating the activity of other genes. Homeotic genes code for the production of a regulatory protein that can bind to DNA and thus affect the transcription of one or more genes. This enables homeotic genes to initiate or halt the development and specialization of characteristics in an organism.

Nearly identical homeotic genes have been identified in varied organisms, such as insects, worms, mice, birds, and humans, where they serve similar embryonic development functions. Scientists theorize that homeotic genes first appeared in a single ancestor common to all these organisms. Sometime in evolutionary history, these organisms diverged from their common ancestor, but the homeotic genes continued to be passed down through generations virtually unchanged during the evolution of these new organisms.

INFORMATION IN DNA AND RNA TRANSLATED TO PROTEIN

How is the information in DNA and RNA translated to protein sequence? A complex machine composed of proteins and ncRNAs called the *ribosome* reads an mRNA sequence and writes a protein sequence. The mRNA is read three nucleotides at a time. The nucleotide triplets are called *codons*. Each codon corresponds to a single amino acid. The mapping from codons to amino acids is called the *genetic code*, and its discovery is one of the great achievements in molecular biology. The genetic code is one of the universal laws of molecular biology (and, as you should expect, is sometimes broken).

Because codons are three nucleotides long and there are four possible nucleotides at each position, it follows that there are 64 (4^3) possible codons. However, there are only 20 amino acids. Thus there is redundancy in the genetic code and in turn, the code is often described as degenerate. Figure shows the standard nuclear genetic code (there are more than a dozen different genetic codes, mostly from different mitochondrial genomes). If you look closely at the redundancies, you will find patterns. For example, the third position of a codon is often insignificant; A, C, G, or T all lead to the same translation. When this isn't the case, A and G are usually synonymous, as are C and T. It so happens that A and G belong to the same chemical class, called *purines,* and C and T belong to another class, called *pyrimidines,* so this makes sense in a biochemical way. There are other neat patterns, such as any codon with a T in the middle translates to a hydrophobic amino acid. In addition to the amino acids, there are three *stop codons*. When a ribosome sees a stop codon, translation terminates, and the protein is released to go about its business. As mentioned before, all proteins start with the amino acid methionine. This has only one codon, ATG, and so ATG is often called the *start codon*.

Consider the following nucleotide sequence:

TTTATATCACAC

If you translate this from the first letter, you get the protein sequence:

FISH

But what if you translate it from the second nucleotide? You get a different protein sequence (note that the fractional codon AC at the end of the DNA translates to threonine no matter what the next nucleotide is):

LYHT

Because codons are three nucleotides long, you can translate DNA in three different *reading frames*. Since DNA is double stranded, there are really six reading frames for every piece of DNA. So if someone hands you a DNA sequence and asks you to translate it, you may have a little trouble.

EVOLUTION

BLAST works because evolution is happening. Biological sequences show complex patterns of similarity to one another. In this regard, they mirror the external morphologies of the organisms in which they reside. You'll notice that birds, for example, show natural groupings.

You don't have to be a biologist to see that ducks, geese, and swans comprise a reasonably natural group called the waterfowl, and that the similarities between ducks and geese seem too great to explain by mere coincidence.

Biological sequences are no different. After all, the reason why ducks look like ducks and geese look like geese is because of their genes. Many molecular biologists are convinced that understanding sequence evolution is tantamount to understanding evolution itself.

Sequences change over time due to three forces: mutation, natural selection, and genetic drift. If you use BLAST, it's important to understand these forces because they form the biological foundation of similarity searches. The biological and mathematical foundations aren't the same, and are sometimes at odds. You need to understand both theories in order to knowledgeably interpret the sequence alignments in a BLAST report.

Mutation

A *mutation* is simply a change in a DNA sequence. What causes mutation? Many chemicals and conditions damage DNA, so its sequence either changes or ceases to be recognizable. Mutagenic agents are often called *carcinogens* because cancer is caused by the accumulation of mutations in genes that control cell division. But even in a world without carcinogens there would still be mutation because the process of DNA replication isn't perfect. Every time a cell divides, it must duplicate its DNA.

The human genome is about three billion letters long, and the error rate of DNA replication is about one error in every 300 million letters, so you can expect about 10 mutations per genome duplication. Genome size varies, as does the replication error rate, so don't take the 10 mutations per genome replication as any kind of biological truth. Human beings are composed of about a trillion cells, and you might take a moment now and consider just how much mutation is going on in your own body. Whatever that large number is, it's infinitesimal compared to what's happening in the biosphere as a whole.

What happens when a mutation occurs in the protein-coding portion of a gene? Because the DNA is mutated, the mRNA is also mutated. This in turn *may* lead to a different protein, but not necessarily, because the genetic code is degenerate. Take a look at an example for which you mutate just one letter in a coding sequence. If the mutation changed a codon from TTA to TTG, for example, the protein would be unchanged because both codons translate to the amino acid leucine. Such mutations are called *silent, synonymous,* or *same-sense* because they don't affect the protein sequence in any way. If the mutation changed a TTA to a TTT, however, the codon would code for a different amino acid, phenylalanine.

Such substitutions are called *mis-sense* mutations. Molecular biologists will often classify mis-sense mutations into either conservative or nonconservative substitutions, depending on whether the two amino acids are chemically similar to one another. Leucine and phenylalanine are both hydrophobic amino acids, and such a substitution would be considered conservative. Bioinformaticists, however, give a more rigorous and quantifiable definition of conservative. If the TTA codon is mutated to TAA, the codon becomes a stop codon, which causes the ribosome to stop translating the mRNA. This represents the most destructive kind of mutation, and is called a *non-sense* mutation. Non-sense mutations cause translation to terminate prematurely, and the result is a truncated protein that may function partially, not function at all, or be poisonous to the cell.

Not all mutations substitute one nucleotide for another. Some mutations may insert or remove nucleotides. In addition, there are duplications, inversions, and other large-scale rearrangements that destroy genes or even fuse them together. Insertions and deletions are often destructive because they change the reading frame of translation if they aren't additions/subtractions of a multiple of three (a whole codon). After such a *frame-shift mutation*, there are usually several mis-sense mutations caused by the out-of-frame codons, and then a premature stop codon that was not previously in frame. Insertions and deletions are therefore usually as disruptive as mis-sense mutations.

What happens to an organism with mutations? It depends on a lot of factors. A mutation may have disastrous consequences, it might prove beneficial, or it might have no effect at all. To understand the forces that govern sequence evolution, let's take a close look at natural selection and genetic drift.

Natural Selection

The theory of natural selection was developed to explain why organisms look the way they do and why they seem to "fit" their environments so well. For example, why do giraffes have such long necks? Historically, there have been a lot of explanations, but we'll skip those debates and focus on the theory of natural selection because it is simple and fits the data well. The theory has only three assumptions.

- There must be variation within a population.
- The variation must be heritable.
- There must be differential reproduction based on variation.

In the case of the giraffe ancestor, those individuals with slightly longer necks were at an advantage because they could reach leaves higher in the trees. This advantage translates to more surviving offspring, and since the variation is heritable, they too will tend to have longish necks. Now, within this population of longish necked pre-giraffes, there is still more variation, and the cycle of selecting for longer-necked individuals can persist until you have something that looks like a modern giraffe. People often look at the organisms today and think that their form is "complete". But all organisms are undergoing change from one generation to the next. When you look at a giraffe, try thinking about it as a particular form at a snapshot in time, on its way to something perhaps taller, or shorter, or with wings and horns and a penchant for breathing fire.

When Charles Darwin formulated the theory of natural selection, he had no idea about mutations, DNA, proteins, or the genetic code. The theory was based solely on observation; there was no known mechanism. In the last 50 years, the advances in molecular biology have revolutionized our understanding of natural selection. We now understand why there is variation and what is being selected for and against. The *why* is that variation exists at the DNA level (called *alleles* by geneticists). The *what* is differences in genes.

Consider how protein structure is selected for or against. What if a mutation causes an amino acid in the hydrophobic core of a protein to be changed to something hydrophilic? Well, it probably wouldn't fold the same way anymore because the hydrophobic core of the globular structure now has a part that wants to be in an aqueous environment. In most cases, changes in protein structure are unfavourable and therefore selected against; however, sometimes they result in altered function, which is favourable in certain conditions. Such is the case with sickle cell anemia. A charged amino acid (glutamate) is changed to a hydrophobic one (valine), causing altered protein interactions at the surface. Disease results when both alleles of the gene have this change, but it offers some protection against malaria when present in only one allele. As natural selection would predict, the sickle cell allele, and therefore sickle cell anemia, is prominent in certain parts of the world where malaria is common.

Several take-home messages are worth stating quite clearly. First, there is an *inexhaustible* source of variation because mutation is constantly happening. Natural selection isn't going to run out of variation. Evolution isn't going to stop. Second, a mutation can't be declared either good or bad on its own. Even a mutation that introduces a stop codon can be beneficial. Look at seedless oranges. It might seem an abomination of nature that they can't reproduce by themselves, but it is this very fact that makes humans breed them. To the seedless orange, genes that allow seeds to form are the kiss of death.

Genetic Drift

The interplay between mutation and natural selection that was just outlined makes a nice story. Like most stories, though, the truth is a lot more complicated. Reading the previous section, you may have concluded that natural selection is an all-powerful force, responsible for determining every nucleotide in a DNA sequence. In such a world, you would expect proteins to be perfectly functioning machines and the DNA sequences that encode them to be the best possible sequence for the job. This might be true in a mathematical model involving infinite population size and limitless generations, but the real biological world is a harsh place subject to happenstance.

Even if the highly advantageous mutation enabling X-ray vision were to arise in some individual, it might not end up in the gene pool if that person thinks he's Superman and tries to stop a runaway train.

Darwin was not aware of how variation is transmitted from generation to generation; he didn't have the concept of genes. Genes were introduced by Gregor Mendel to explain how hereditary information is transmitted from one generation to the next. Combining Mendelian genetics and natural selection led to the field of population genetics, which is chiefly concerned with the changes in allele frequencies over time. Mathematical simulations show quite clearly that allele frequencies can change by purely random processes. This behaviour is called *genetic drift*, and it's based on the fact that populations aren't infinitely large.

Let's demonstrate genetic drift with an example. For simplicity, let's ignore new mutations and just consider an anonymoussite that has no consequence in natural selection. Assume there are only 10 individuals in the population, and that 5 have a C at this position and 5 have a T. Keeping the population fixed, in the next generation, the allele frequencies may change to C=0.6 and T=0.4 due to a runaway train or, less spectacularly, sampling error. All things being equal, in the next generation, there's a greater chance that the C will increase and the T will decrease. If this trend continues for a few generations, the T's may disappear from the population entirely at which point the C allele is considered *fixed* in the population. Alleles can be fixed very rapidly if some individuals move away to form a new population. This is called the *founder effect*. As you can see, changes in allele frequencies don't require mutation or natural selection.

RESTRICTION MODIFICATION SYSTEM

Phage (or viruses) invade all types of cells. Bacteria are one favourite target. Defense mechanisms have been developed by bacteria to defend themselves from these invasions.

The system they possess for this defence is the restriction-modificiation system. This system is composed of a restriction endonuclease enzyme and a methylase enzyme and each bacterial species and strain has their own combination of restriction and methylating enzymes.

Restriction Enzyme

An enzyme that cuts DNA at internal phosphodiester bonds; different types exist and the most useful ones for molecular biology (Type II) are those which cleave at a specific DNA sequence

Methylase

An enzyme that adds a methyl group to a molecule; in restriction-modification systems of bacteria a methyl group is added to DNA at a specific site to protect the site from restriction endonuclease cleavage Several different types of restriction enzymes have been found but the most useful ones for molecular biology and genetic engineering are the Type II restriction enzymes. These enzymes cut DNA at specific nucleotide sequences. For example, the enzyme EcoRI recognises the sequence:

$$5' - G A A^* T T C - 3'$$

$$3' - C T T^* A A G - 5'$$

The site of methylation protection from restriction enzyme cleavage is the 3' adenine. This enzyme always cuts between the 5' G and A residues. But if we look at the sequence we can see that both strands will be cut and leave staggered or overlapping ends.

$$5' - G A A T T C - 3'$$

$$3' - C T T A A G - 5'$$

Not all Type II restriction enzymes generate staggered ends at the target site. Some cut and leave blunt ends. For example, the enzyme BalI.

$$5' - T G G C^* C A - 3'$$

$$3' - A C^* C G G T - 5'$$

is cut at the point of symmetry to produce:

$$5' - T G G C C A - 3'$$

$$3' - A C C G G T - 5'$$

Note: The site of methylation protection from restriction enzyme cleavage; 5' cytosine.

We began this discussion by stating that the restriction-modification system is used to protect bacteria from invasion by viral DNA molecules that may subvert the gene expression system of the bacteria to its own use. But how does this system actually work? The bacterial cell uses the restriction enzyme to cut the invading DNA of the virus at the specific recognition site of the enzyme. This prevents the virus from taking over the cellular metabolism for its own replication. But bacterial DNA will also contain sites that could be cleaved by the restriction enzyme. How is the bacterial cell protected? This protection is offered by the action of the methylase. The methylase recognises the same target site as the restriction enzyme and adds a methyl group to a specific nucleotide in the restriction site. Methylated sites are not substrates for the restriction enzyme. The bacterial DNA is methylated immediately following replication so it will not be a suitable substrate for restriction endonuclease cleavage. But it is unlikely that the invading viral DNA will have been methylated so it will be an appropriate target for cleavage. Thus, the viral DNA is *restricted* in the bacterial cell by the restriction enzyme, and the bacterial DNA is *modified* by the methylase and is provided protection from its own restriction enzyme.

Methylation of Plant DNA and Its Effect on Restriction Digestion

The following discussion is based on the experiments described by Grenbaum *et al.* in the paper "Methylation of Cytosines in Higher Plants". The paper was published in Nature 297:86 August 1981. It was noted that 5-methyl cytosine (5mC) is found to be a component of plant DNA much more frequently than animal DNA. The following table shows the distribution.

	per cent Cytosine as 5mC
Animals	2-7
Plants	>25

What is the experimental explanation for such a high level of 5mC?

- 5mC occurs at 70-80 per cent of the 5'-CG-3' dinucleotides. What are the occurrences of the dinucleotide in the two kingdoms?

	% dinucleotides as 5-'CG-3
Animals	0.5-1.0
Plants	3.4

- 5mC also occurs at the 5'-CXG-3' sequence in plants but does not occur in animals. How often are these sequences methylated in plants?

Sequence	% C methylated
5'-CAG-3'	80
5'-CCG-3'	50

What ramifications does this have for performing restriction digests of plant? Restriction digestion and subsequent hybridisations are important for genomic and RFLP analysis of plants. For this analysis to be informative, the

DNA must be digested to completion. Thus it is important to chose the correct enzymes for analysis. Because plant DNA is highly C-methylated, it is important to chose an enzyme for digestion experiments that are not affected by C-methylation.

Do Not Use These Enzymes to Analyse Plant DNA

- Restriction site has 5'-CXG-3'

Enzyme Site	Sequence
PstI	5'-C*TGCAG-3'
PvuII	5'-CAGC*TG-3'
MspI	5'-C*CGG-3
EcoRII	5'-CC*WGG-3' (W = A or T)

(Base preceeding the * is methylated.)

- C at or near end of site;if next base in DNA is G, it will be methylated

Enzyme	Site Sequence
BamHI	5'-GGATC*C-3
KpnI	5'-GGTACC*-3

(Base preceeding the * is methylated.)

Use These Enzymes Instead to Cut Plant DNA

Enzyme	Site Sequence
DraI	5'-TTTAAA-3'
EcoRV	5-'GA*TATC-3
EcoRI	5-GAA*TTC*-3'
HindIII	5'-A*AGC*TT-3'
XbaI	5'-TC*TAGA*-3'

(Base preceeding the * is methylated.)

Nucleic Acid Hybridisations

The hybridisation of a radioactive probe to filter bound DNA or RNA is one of the most informative experiments that is performed in molecular genetics.

Two basic types of hybridisations are possible:

1. *Southern hybridisation*: Hybridisation of a probe to filter bound DNA; the DNA is typically transferred to the filter from a gel
2. *Northern hybridisation*: Hybridisation of a probe to filter bound RNA; the RNA is typically transferred to the filter from a gel

Probes are the primary tool used to identify complementary sequences of interest. Generally, the probe is a clone developed by inserting DNA into a vector. Most often these are plasmid clones.

- *Probe*: A single-stranded nucleic acid that has been radiolabelled and is used to identify a complimentary nucleic acid sequence that is membrane bound

The hyrbridisation process involves two different steps. First the nucleic acid must be immobilised on a filter. This is generally called a "Southern Transfer" procedure. The second step is the actual hybridisation of the probe to the filter bound nucleic acid.

The following steps describe the Southern transfer procedure:

- Digest DNA with the restriction enzyme of choice.
- Load the digestion onto a agarose gel and apply an electrical current. DNA is negatively charged so it migrates towards the "+" pole. The distance a specific fragment migrates is inversely proportional to the fragment size.
- Stain the gel with EtBr, a fluorescent dye which intercalates into the DNA molecule. The DNA can be visualised with a UV light source to assess the completeness of the digestion.
- Denature the double-stranded fragments by soaking the gel in alkali (>0.4 M NaOH).
- Transfer the DNA to a filter membrane (nylon or nitrocellulose) by capillary action. Typically a Southern transferst setup contains (from bottom to top):
  - Buffer
  - Sponge
  - Filter paper
  - The gel containing the nucleic acid
  - A nylon or nitrocellulose membrane
  - More filter paper
  - Paper towels to catch the buffer that passed through all of the above

Southern hybridisations with plant DNA is not a trivial matter. The primary requirement for a successful experiment is that the DNA to be probed is digested to completion. We have already discussed the choice of enzymes in this regard. Even when using compatible enzymes (not GC or GXC sensitive) monitoring the completeness of the reaction is essential for consistent results. Once you are satisfied that you completely digested the DNA and are confident that it was successfully transferred to the filter membrane, the next step is perform the actual hybridisation. The following steps describe the procedure.

Steps in Southern Hybridisation Procedure

- Prepare a probe by nick translation or random, oligo-primed labelling.
- Add the probe to a filter (nylon or nitrocellulose) to which single-stranded nucleic acids are bound. (The filter is protected with a prehybridisation solution which contains molecules which fill in the spots on the filter where the nucleic acid has not bound.
- Hybridise the single-stranded probe to the filter-bound nucleic acid for 24 hr. The probe will bind to complementary sequences.
- Wash the filter to remove non-specifically bound probe.
- Expose the filter and determine:
  - Did binding occur?
  - If so, what is the size of hybridizing fragment?

Hybridisation Stringency

The temperature and salt concentrations at which we perform a hybridisation has a direct effect upon the results that are obtained. Specifically, you can set the conditions up so that your hybridisations only occur between the probe and a filter bound nucleic acid that is highly homologous to that probe. You can also adjust the conditions the hybridsation is to a nucleic acid that has a lower degree of homology to the probe. Your hybridisation results are directly related to the number of degrees below the Tm of DNA at which the experiment is performed. For a aqueous solution of DNA (no salt) the formula for Tm is:

$$T_m = 69.3°C + 0.41(\% \ G + C)°C$$

From this formula you can see that the GC content has a direct effect on Tm. The following examples, demonstrate the point.

$$T_m = 69.3°C + 0.41(45)°C = 87.5°C \text{ (for wheat germ)}$$
$$T_m = 69.3°C + 0.41(40)°C = 85.7°C$$
$$T_m = 69.3°C + 0.41(60)°C = 93.9°C$$

Hybridisations though are always performed with salt. This requires another formula which that takes the salt concentration into account. Under salt-containing hybridisation conditions, the effective Tm is what controls he degeree of homology between the probe and the filter bound DNA is required for successful hybridisation. The formula for the Effective Tm (Eff T_m).

$$\text{Eff } T_m = 81.5 + 16.6(\log M [Na+]) + 0.41(\%G+C)$$
$$- 0.72(\% \text{ formamide})$$

The salt solution that is most often used in hybridisation experiments is SSC (standard sodium citrate). Different concentrations of this solution are used at different steps in the hybridisation procedure. The following table gives the Na+ concentration for different strengths of SSC. Remember that this value is essential to derive the Eff T_m.

Na+ ion Concentration of Different Strengths of SSC

SSC Content	[Na+] M
20X	3.3000
10X	1.6500
5X	0.8250
2X	0.3300
1X	0.1650
0.1X	0.0165

Another relevant relationship is a that *1 per cent mismatch of two DNAs lowers the T_m 1.4°C*. So in a hybridisation with wheat germ that is performed at T_m - 20°C (=67.5°C), the two DNAs must be 85.7 per cent homologous for the hybridisation to occur. 100 per cent - (20°C/1.4°C) = 85.7 per cent homology. Let's now look at an actual experiment, the hybridisation of a probe with filter bound wheat DNA in 5X SSC at 65°C. The first step is to derive the Eff T_m.

$$\text{Eff } T_m = 81.5 + 16.6(\log 0.825) + 18.5 = 98.6°C$$

These types of hybridisation experiments are typically performed at T_m - 20°C. A typical temperature of hybridisation is 65°C. (If formamide is used the hybridisation is normally performed at 42°C). With these conditions, 83.1 per cent homology between the probe and filter bound DNA is required for hybridisation. The following calculation is how this number was derived.

$$100- [(98.6-65.0)/1.4] = 100 - (23.6/1.4) = 83.1 \text{ per cent.}$$

The next step in a hybridisation experiment is to wash the filter. This is normally done in two steps. First a non-stringent wash is performed to remove the non-specifically bound DNA and the second wash is performed at a higher stringency that only permits highly homologous sequences to remain bound to the filter. Controlling the stringency is an important step in these experiments.

- *Stringency*: A term used in hybridisation experiments to denote the degree of homology between the probe and the filter bound nucleic acid; the higher the stringency, the higher per cent homology between the probe and filter bound nucleic acid
- *Non-stringent wash*: Normally 2X SSC, 65°C

$$\text{Eff } T_m = 81.5 + 16.6[\log(0.33)] + 0.41(45\%) = 92.0°C$$
$$\%\text{Homology} = 100 - [(92-65)/1.4] = 80.7\%$$

- *Stringent wash*: Normally 0.1X SSC, 65°C

$$\text{Eff } T_m = 81.5 + 16.6[\log(0.0165)] + 0.41(45\%) = 70.4°C$$
$$\%\text{Homology} = 100 - [(70.4-65)/1.4] = 96.1\%$$

This example shows that the final wash is the one of concern when determining the relatedness of the probe and the filter bound nucleic acid.

- *An example*: Bowman-Kirk Protease Inhibitor Final wash is performed at 0.2X SSC, 55°C; assume 45% GCcontent

$$\text{Eff } T_m = 81.5 + 16.6[\log(0.033)] + 18.5 = 75.4°C$$
$$\%\text{Homology} = 100 - [(75.4-55.0)/1.4] = 85.4\%$$

The point to this last example to emphasise that your per cent homology is directly related to your most stringent condition in your hybridisation experiment. This invariably is the final wash. Thus, you only need to make this calculation to determine the stringency of your experiment.

Southern Hybridisations

Southern hybridisations have many applications. The first application after cloning a gene is often to determine how many copies of the gene are in the species from which the gene was cloned. This experiment is performed by hybridizing a clone of the gene to total DNA that has been digested with several enzymes. The procedure is termed a *genomic southern.*

One gene that has drawn intense interest because of its potential applied usage in plant biotechnology is chitinase. We have already discussed the isolation of a clone for this gene from bean. As you can imagine, the gene has also been cloned from other species. The first page of hybridisation handout shows the southern hybridisation pattern obtained from cucumber, rice and bean. These hybridisations show that these species contain *different copy numbers* for the gene. A second application for southern hybridisations is the estimation of copy number of a specific gene. This experiment is performed by running several lanes with different copy numbers of the gene to which you are probing and comparing the hybridisation intensities with a companion genomic southern experiment. This is called a*reconstruction experiment.* The example in on the second page of the handout is for phaseolin, the major storage protein of bean. In this example, 1, 2 and 5 genomic equivalents are seen in lanes 7-9. The other lanes are various restriction digestions of total bean DNA. After hybridisation, densitometric readings were taken and it was determined that bean contained 6.5 copies of the gene. This agreed with the data obtained from reassociation kinetic experiments.

Southern hybridisation analysis can also be performed to determine if a phenotypic mutation is due to a structural change in the gene controlling the trait of interest. If a gene undergoes an insertion or deletion the resulting hybridisation pattern would be changed. Insertional mutagenesis would generate fragments of an increased size whereas deletions would reduce the size of the hybridizing band. Two tomato mutants, Neverripe (nr) and ripening inhibitor (ri) express polygalacturonase, an enzyme involved in fruit ripening, at lower levels than normal or wild type tomato. The question posed here was whether the structure of the polygalacturonase (and other ripening specific genes) are structurally different than the wild type genotype. The thrid page of the handout. shows that the structure of these genes in the mutatnt is not different than the wild type. Therefore, some other molecular event is responsible for these differences in expression patterns of the different mutants.

4

Bacteriology

The beginnings of bacteriology paralleled the development of the microscope. The first person to see microorganisms was probably the Dutch naturalist Antonie van Leeuwenhoek, who in 1683 described some animalcules, as they were then called, in water, saliva, and other substances. These had been seen with a simple lens magnifying about 100–150 diameters. The organisms seem to correspond with some of the very large forms of bacteria as now recognized.

As late as the mid-19th century, bacteria were known only to a few experts and in a few forms as curiosities of the microscope, chiefly interesting for their minuteness and motility. Modern understanding of the forms of bacteria dates from Ferdinand Cohn's brilliant classifications, the chief results of which were published at various periods between 1853 and 1872. While Cohn and others advanced knowledge of the morphology of bacteria, other researchers, such as Louis Pasteur andRobert Koch, established the connections between bacteria and the processes of fermentation and disease, in the process discarding the theory of spontaneous generation and improving antisepsis in medical treatment.

The modern methods of bacteriological technique had their beginnings in 1870–85 with the introduction of the use of stains and by the discovery of the method of separating mixtures of organisms on plates of nutrient media solidified with gelatin or agar. Important discoveries came in 1880 and 1881, when Pasteur succeeded in immunizing animals against two diseases caused by bacteria. His research led to a study of disease prevention and the treatment of disease by vaccines and immune serums (a branch of medicine now called immunology). Other scientists recognized the importance of bacteria in agriculture and the dairy industry.

Bacteriological study subsequently developed a number of specializations, among which are agricultural, or soil, bacteriology; clinical diagnostic bacteriology; industrial bacteriology; marine bacteriology; public-health bacteriology; sanitary, or hygienic, bacteriology; and systematic bacteriology, which deals with taxonomy.

GENERAL CONCEPTS OF BRUCELLA

Clinical Manifestations

Brucellosis is a severe acute febrile disease caused by bacteria of the genus Brucella.

- Relapses are not uncommon;
- Focal lesions may occur in bones, joints, genitourinary tract, and other sites.
- Hypersensitivity reactions can follow occupational exposure.
- Infection may be subclinical.
- Chronic infections may occur.

Structure

Brucellae are:

- Gram-negative coccobacilli;
- non-spore-forming and
- non-motile;
- aerobic, but may need added CO2.

Classification and Antigenic Types

Three species (B melitensis, B abortus, B suis) are important human pathogens; B canis is of lesser importance. Species are differentiated by

- Production of urease and H2S,
- Dye sensitivity,
- Cell wall antigens and
- Phage sensitivity.

The major species are divided into multiple biovars.

Pathogenesis

Portals of entry are the mouth, conjunctivae, respiratory tract and abraded skin. Organisms spread, possibly in mononuclear phagocytes, to reticuloendothelial sites. Small granulomas reveal a mononuclear response; hypersensitivity is a major factor.

Host Defences

Effective host defence depends mainly upon cell-mediated immunity.

Epidemiology

Brucellosis is a zoonosis, acquired from

- Handling of infected animals or
- Consuming contaminated milk or milk products.

Exposure is frequently occupational. The disease is now uncommon in the United States and Britain but common in the Mediterranean and Arabian Gulf regions, Latin America, Africa, and parts of Asia.

Diagnosis

Diagnosis can be made clinically if there is a history of exposure. Blood cultures may be positive in early disease but serology is mainstay of diagnosis. Interpretation is complicated by subclinical infections and persistent levels of antibody.

Control

Brucellosis is prevented by

- Pasteurizing milk,
- Eradicating infection from herds and flocks, and
- Observing safety precautions (protective clothing and laboratory containment).

The disease is treated with doxycycline, streptomycin and rifampin.

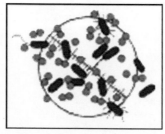

IDENTIFICATION OF BACTERIA

Classic Methods

The criteria used for microscopic identification of procaryotes include cell shape and grouping, Gram-stain reaction, and motility. Bacterial cells almost invariably take one of three forms: rod (bacillus), sphere (coccus), or spiral (spirillaand spirochetes). Rods that are curved are called vibrios. Fixed bacterial cells stain either Gram-positive (purple) or Gram-negative (pink); motility is easily determined by observing living specimens.

Bacilli may occur singly or form chains of cells; cocci may form chains (streptococci) or grape-like clusters (staphylococci); spiral shape cells are almost always motile; cocci are almost never motile. This nomenclature ignores the actinomycetes, a prominent group of branched bacteria which occur in the soil. But they are easily recognized by their colonies and their microscopic appearance.

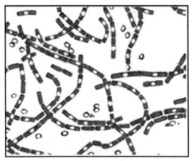

Fig. Gram Stain of **Bacillus Anthracis,** the *Cause of Anthrax*

Such easily-made microscopic observations, combined with knowing the natural environment of the organism, are important aids to identify the group, if not the exact genus, of a bacterium - providing, of course, that one has an effective key. Such a key is Bergey's Manual of Determinative Bacteriology 9th ed, the "field guide" to identification of the bacteria. Bergey's Manual describes affiliated groups of Bacteria and Archaea based on a few easily observed microscopic and physiologic characteristics. Further identification requires biochemical tests which will distinguish genera among families and species among genera. Strains within a single species are usually distinguished by genetic or immunological criteria.

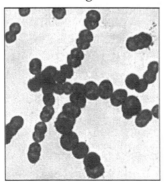

Fig. Streptococcus pyogenes by Maria Fazio and Vincent A. Fischetti, Ph.D. with Permission

Molecular Techniques

The sciences of genomics and bioinformatics have led to a radical reclassification of procaryotes based on comparative analysis of organismal DNA. Genomics involves the study of all of the nucleotide sequences, including structural genes, regulatory sequences, and non-coding DNA segments, in the chromosomes of an organism. To date over 200 bacterial genomes have been sequenced. We have seen how highly conserved genetic sequences, such as those that encode for the small subunit ribosomal RNAs (16S rRNA) of an organism, can be analyzed to specifically relate two organisms. So can the identification of certain genes provide information about specific properties of an organism, and analysis of specific nucleotide sequences may be used to indicate identity and degrees of genetic relatedness among organisms.

The newest editions of Bergey's Manual are adapted to the new phylogenetic classification. This has resulted in the formation of several new taxa of bacteria and archaea at every hierarchical level. Occasionally, organisms thought to be more or less distantly related become unified; but more likely, organisms thought to be closely-related due to similar phenotypic properties are found to be genetically distinct and warrant separation into a new taxa.

Metagenomics. Sequencing of 16S rRNA genes obtained from environmental samples produces a broad profile of microbial diversity and reveals that the vast majority of microbes present have been missed by reliance on cultivation-based methods. This observation has given rise to the field of metagenomics. Metagenomics (also called environmental genomics) is the application of modern genomics techniques to the study of communities of microorganisms directly in their natural environments, bypassing the need for isolation and lab cultivation of individual species. Metagenomics provides a means to identify and quantify microbes from environmental samples based on the presence of distinctive genes. This enables studies of organisms that are not easily cultured in the laboratory, as well as studies of organisms in their natural environment.

"Shotgun" metagenomics is capable of sequencing nearly complete microbial genomes directly from the environment. Because the collection of DNA from an environment is largely uncontrolled, the most abundant organisms in a sample are most highly represented in the resulting sequence data. To achieve the high coverage needed to fully resolve the genomes of underrepresented community members, large samples, often prohibitively so, may be needed. However, the random nature of shotgun sequencing ensures that many of these organisms will be represented by at least some small sequence segments. Due to the limitations of microbial isolation methods, the majority of these organisms would go unnoticed using traditional culturing techniques. Shotgun sequencing and screens of clone libraries reveal genes present in environmental samples. This provides information both on which organisms are present and what metabolic processes are possible in the community. This can be helpful in understanding the ecology of a community, particularly if multiple samples are compared to one other.

ECOLOGY OF BACTERIA AND ARCHAEA

Bacteria and Archaea are present in all environments that support life. They may be free-living, or living in associations with "higher forms" of life (plants and animals), and they are found in environments that support no other form of life. Procaryotes have the usual nutritional requirements for growth of cells, but many of the ways that they utilize and transform their nutrients are unique. This bears directly on their habitat and their ecology.

Nutritional Types of Organisms

In terms of carbon utilization a cell may be heterotrophic or autotrophic.Heterotrophs obtain their carbon and energy for growth from organic compounds in nature. Autotrophs use CO_2 as a sole source of carbon for growth and obtain their energy from light (*e.g.* photoautotrophs) or from the oxidation of inorganic compounds (*e.g.* lithoautotrophs).

Most heterotrophic bacteria are saprophytes, meaning that they obtain their nourishment from dead organic matter. In the soil, saprophytic bacteria and fungi are responsible for biodegradation of organic material. Ultimately, organic molecules, no matter how complex, can be degraded to CO_2 (plus H_2 and H_2O). Probably no naturally-occurring organic substance cannot be degraded by the combined activities of the bacteria and fungi. Hence, most organic matter in nature is converted by heterotrophs to CO_2, only to be converted back into organic material by autotrophs that die and nourish heterotrophs to complete the carbon cycle.

Lithotrophic procaryotes have a type of energy-producing metabolism which is unique. Lithotrophs (also called lithoautotrophs or chemoautotrophs) use inorganic compounds as sources of energy, *i.e.*, they oxidize compounds such as H_2 or H_2S or NH_3 to obtain electrons to feed in to an electron transport system and to produce ATP. Lithotrophs are found in soil and aquatic environments wherever their energy source is present. Most lithotrophs are autotrophs so they can grow in the absence of any organic material. Lithotrophic species are found among the Bacteria and the Archaea. Sulfur-oxidizing lithotrophs convert H_2S to S^o and S^o to SO_4. Nitrifying bacteria convert NH_3 to NO_2 and NO_2 to NO_3; methanogenic archaea strip electrons off of H_2 as a source of energy and add them to CO_2 to form CH_4 (methane). Lithotrophs have an obvious impact on the sulfur, nitrogen and carbon cycles in the biosphere. Photosynthetic bacteria convert light energy into chemical energy for growth. Most phototrophic bacteria are autotrophs so their role in the carbon cycle is analogous to that of plants. The planktonic cyanobacteria are the "grass of the sea" and their form of oxygenic photosynthesis generates a substantial amount of O_2 in the biosphere. However, among the photosynthetic bacteria are types of photosynthetic metabolism not seen in eucaryotes, includingphotoheterotrophy (using light as an energy source while assimilating organic compounds as a source of carbon), anoxygenic photosynthesis, and unique mechanisms of CO_2 fixation (autotrophy).

Photosynthesis has not been found to occur among the Archaea, but one archaeal species employs a light-driven non- photosynthetic means of energy generation based on the use of a chromophore called bacteriorhodopsin.

Adaptations to Environmental Conditions

Most procaryotes, whether they have been cultured and studied in the laboratory, or observed growing in their natural habitats, seem to be highly adapted to their specific environment by means of their macromolecular structure and/or their physiologic (metabolic) capabilities. The nutritional quality of the environment determines whether a particular organism will be present, but so do various physical parameters such as the availability of light and O_2, as well as the pH, temperature and salinity of the environment. As examples, the range of procaryotic responses to oxygen and temperature are discussed below.

Procaryotes vary widely in their response to O_2 (molecular oxygen). Organisms that require O_2 for growth are called obligate aerobes; those which are inhibited or killed by O_2, and which grow only in its absence, are called obligate anaerobes; organisms which grow either in the presence or absence of O_2 are called facultative anaerobes. Whether or not a particular organism can exist in the presence of O_2 depends upon the distribution of certain enzymes such as superoxide dismutase and catalase that are required to detoxify lethal oxygen radicals that are always generated by living systems in the presence of O_2

Procaryotes also vary widely in their response to temperature. Those that live at very cold temperatures (0 degrees or lower) are called psychrophiles; those which flourish at room temperature (25 degrees) or at the temperature of warm-blooded animals (37 degrees) are called mesophiles; those that live at high temperatures (greater than 45 degrees) are thermophiles. The only limit that seems to be placed on growth of certain procaryotes in nature relative to temperature is whether liquid water exists.

Hence, growing procaryotic cells can be found in supercooled environments (ice does not form) as low as -20 degrees and superheated environments (steam does not form) as high as 120 degrees. Archaea have been detected around thermal vents on the ocean floor where the temperature is as high as 320 degrees!

Symbiosis

The biomass of procaryotic cells in the biosphere, their metabolic diversity, and their persistence in all habitats that support life, ensures that these microbe will play a crucial role in the cycles of elements and the functioning of the world ecosystem. However, the procaryotes affect the world ecology in another significant way through their inevitable interactions with insects, plants and animals.

Some bacteria are required to associate with insects, animals or plants for the latter to survive. For example, the sex of offspring of certain insects is determined by endosymbiotic bacteria. Ruminant animals (cows, sheep, etc.), whose diet is mainly cellulose (plant material), must have cellulose-digesting bacteria in their intestine to convert the cellulose to a form of carbon that the animal can assimilate. Leguminous plants grow poorly in nitrogen-deprived soils unless they are colonized by nitrogen-fixing bacteria which can supply them with a biologically-useful form of nitrogen.

Bacterial Pathogenicity

Some bacteria are parasites of plants or animals, meaning that they grow at the expense of their eucaryotic host and may damage, harm, or even kill it in the process. Such bacteria that cause disease in plants or animals arepathogens.

Human diseases caused by bacterial pathogens include tuberculosis, whooping cough, diphtheria, tetanus, gonorrhea, syphilis, pneumonia, cholera and typhoid fever, to name a few. The bacteria that cause these diseases have special structural or biochemical properties that determine their virulence or pathogenicity. These include: (1) ability to colonize and invade their host; (2) ability to resist or withstand the antibacterial defences of the host; (3) ability to produce various toxic substances that damage the host. Plant diseases, likewise, may be caused by bacterial pathogens. More than 200 species of bacteria are associated with plant diseases, but a very small handful of genera are involved.

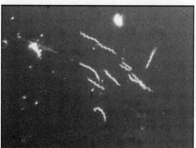

Fig. **Borrelia burgdorferi.** *This spirochete is the bacterial parasite that causes Lyme disease*

MEASUREMENT OF BACTERIAL GROWTH

Growth is an orderly increase in the quantity of cellular constituents. It depends upon the ability of the cell to form new protoplasm from nutrients available in the environment. In most bacteria, growth involves increase in cell mass and number of ribosomes, duplication of the bacterial chromosome, synthesis of new cell wall and plasma membrane, partitioning of the two chromosomes, septum formation, and cell division. This asexual process of reproduction is called binary fission.

Methods for Measurement of Cell Numbers

Measuring techniques involve direct counts, visually or instrumentally, and indirect viable cell counts.

- Direct microscopic counts are possible using special slides known as counting chambers. Dead cells cannot be distinguished from living ones. Only dense suspensions can be counted (>10^7 cells per ml), but samples can be concentrated by centrifugation or filtration to increase sensitivity.

  A variation of the direct microscopic count has been used to observe and measure growth of bacteria in natural environments. In order to detect and prove that thermophilic bacteria were growing in boiling hot springs, T.D. Brock immersed microscope slides in the springs and withdrew them periodically for microscopic observation. The bacteria in the boiling water attached to the glass slides naturally and grew as microcolonies on the surface.

- Electronic counting chambers count numbers and measure size distribution of cells. For cells the size of bacteria the suspending medium must be very clean. Such electronic devices are more often used to count eucaryotic cells such as blood cells.

- Indirect viable cell counts, also called plate counts, involve plating out (spreading) a sample of a culture on a nutrient agar surface. The sample or cell suspension can be diluted in a non-toxic diluent (*e.g.* water or saline) before plating. If plated on a suitable medium, each viable unit grows and forms a colony. Each colony that can be counted is called a colony forming unit (cfu)and the number of cfu's is related to the viable number of bacteria in the sample.

Advantages of the technique are its sensitivity (theoretically, a single cell can be detected), and it allows for inspection and positive identification of the organism counted. Disadvantages are:

- Only living cells develop colonies that are counted;
- Clumps or chains of cells develop into a single colony;
- Colonies develop only from those organisms for which the cultural conditions are suitable for growth.

The latter makes the technique virtually useless to characterize or count the total number of bacteria in complex microbial ecosystems such as soil or the animal rumen or gastrointestinal tract. Genetic probes can be used to demonstrate the diversity and relative abundance of procaryotes in such an environment, but many species identified by genetic techniques have so far proven unculturable.

The Bacterial Growth Curve

In the laboratory, under favourable conditions, a growing bacterial population doubles at regular intervals. Growth is by geometric progression: 1, 2, 4, 8, etc. or 2^0, 2^1, 2^2, 2^3.........2^n (where n = the number of generations). This is calledexponential growth. In reality, exponential growth is only part of the bacterial life cycle, and not representative of the normal pattern of growth of bacteria in Nature. When a fresh medium is inoculated with a given number of cells, and the population growth is monitored over a period of time, plotting the data will yield atypical bacterial growth curve.

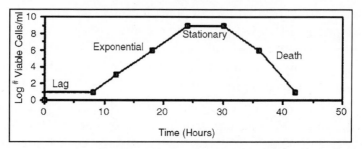

Fig. The typical bacterial growth curve. When bacteria are grown in a closed system, like a test tube, the population of cells almost always exhibits these growth dynamics: cells initially adjust to the new medium until they can start dividing regularly by the process of binary fission (exponential phase)

Four characteristic phases of the growth cycle are recognized:

1. Lag Phase. Immediately after inoculation of the cells into fresh medium, the population remains temporarily unchanged. Although there is no apparent cell division occurring, the cells may be growing in volume or mass, synthesizing enzymes, proteins, RNA, etc., and increasing in metabolic activity.

   The length of the lag phase is apparently dependent on a wide variety of factors including the size of the inoculum; time necessary to recover from physical damage or shock in the transfer; time required for synthesis of essential coenzymes or division factors; and time required for synthesis of new (inducible) enzymes that are necessary to metabolize the substrates present in the medium.

2. Exponential (log) Phase. The exponential phase of growth is a pattern of balanced growth wherein all the cells are dividing regularly by binary fission, and are growing by geometric progression. The cells divide at a constant rate depending upon the composition of the growth medium and the conditions of incubation. The rate of exponential growth of a bacterial culture is expressed asgeneration time, also the doubling time of the bacterial population. Generation time (G) is defined as the time (t) per generation (n = number of generations). Hence, $G=t/n$ is the equation from which calculations of generation time (below) derive.

3. Stationary Phase. Exponential growth cannot be continued forever in abatch culture (*e.g.* a closed system such as a test tube or flask). Population growth is limited by one of three factors: 1. exhaustion of available nutrients; 2. accumulation of inhibitory metabolites or end

products; 3. exhaustion of space, in this case called a lack of "biological space".

During the stationary phase, if viable cells are being counted, it cannot be determined whether some cells are dying and an equal number of cells are dividing, or the population of cells has simply stopped growing and dividing. The stationary phase, like the lag phase, is not necessarily a period of quiescence. Bacteria that produce secondary metabolites, such as antibiotics, do so during the stationary phase of the growth cycle (Secondary metabolites are defined as metabolites produced after the active stage of growth). It is during the stationary phase that spore-forming bacteria have to induce or unmask the activity of dozens of genes that may be involved in sporulation process.

4. Death Phase. If incubation continues after the population reaches stationary phase, a death phase follows, in which the viable cell population declines. (Note, if counting by turbidimetric measurements or microscopic counts, the death phase cannot be observed.). During the death phase, the number of viable cells decreases geometrically (exponentially), essentially the reverse of growth during the log phase.

Growth Rate and Generation Time

As mentioned above, bacterial growth rates during the phase of exponential growth, under standard nutritional conditions (culture medium, temperature, pH, etc.), define the bacterium's generation time. Generation times for bacteria vary from about 12 minutes to 24 hours or more. The generation time for *E. coli* in the laboratory is 15-20 minutes, but in the intestinal tract, the coliform's generation time is estimated to be 12-24 hours. For most known bacteria that can be cultured, generation times range from about 15 minutes to 1 hour. Symbionts such as *Rhizobium* tend to have longer generation times. Many lithotrophs, such as the nitrifying bacteria, also have long generation times. Some bacteria that are pathogens, such as *Mycobacterium tuberculosis* and *Treponema pallidum*, have especially long generation times, and this is thought to be an advantage in their virulence. Generation times for a few bacteria.

SYNCHRONOUS GROWTH OF BACTERIA

Studying the growth of bacterial populations in batch or continuous cultures does not permit any conclusions about the growth behaviour of individual cells, because the distribution of cell size (and hence cell age) among the members of the population is completely random. Information about the growth behaviour of individual bacteria can, however, be obtained by the study of synchronous cultures. Synchronized cultures must be composed of cells which are all at the same stage of the bacterial cell cycle. Measurements made on synchronized cultures are equivalent to measurements made on individual cells.

A number of clever techniques have been devised to obtain bacterial populations at the same stage in the cell cycle. Some techniques involve manipulation of environmental parameters which induces the population to start or stop growth at the same point in the cell cycle, while others are physical methods for selection of cells that have just completed the process of binary fission. Theoretically, the smallest cells in a bacterial population are those that have just completed the process of cell division. Synchronous growth of a population of bacterial cells is illustrated in Figure. Synchronous cultures rapidly lose synchrony because not all cells in the population divide at exactly the same size, age or time.

BACTERIA OF THE GENUS BRUCELLA CAUSE DISEASE

Bacteria of the genus Brucella cause disease primarily in domestic, feral and some wild animals and most are also pathogenic for humans. In animals, brucellae typically affect the reproductive organs, and abortion is often the only sign of the disorder. Human brucellosis is either an acute febrile disease or a persistent disease with a wide variety of symptoms.

It is a true zoonosis in that virtually all human infections are acquired from animals. The disease is controlled by the routine practice of pasteurizing milk and milk products, as well as by comprehensive campaigns to eradicate the disease by destroying domestic animals which exhibit positive serologic reactions to brucellae. Vaccines providing some protection to cattle, sheep and goats are available.

Clinical Manifestations

The presentation of brucellosis is characteristically variable. The incubation period is often difficult to determine but is usually from 2 to 4 weeks. The onset may be insidious or abrupt. Subclinical infection is common. In the simplest case, the

- Onset is influenzalike with fever reaching 38 to 40oC.
- Limb and back pains are unusually severe, however,
- And sweating and fatigue are marked.

- The leukocyte count tends to be normal or reduced, with a relative lymphocytosis. On physical examination,
- Splenomegaly may be the only finding.

If the disease is not treated, the symptoms may continue for 2 to 4 weeks. Many patients will then recover spontaneously but others may suffer a series of exacerbations. These may produce an undulant fever in which the intensity of fever and symptoms recur and recede at about 10 day intervals. Anemia is often a feature. True relapses may occur months after the initial episode, even after apparently successful treatment.

- Most affected persons recover entirely within 3 to 12 months but
- Some will develop complications marked by involvement of various organs, and
- A few may enter an ill-defined chronic syndrome.

Complications include

- Arthritis, often sacroiliitis, and spondylitis (in about 10 per cent of cases),
- Central nervous system effects including meningitis (in about 5 per cent),
- Uveitis and,
- Occasionally, epididymoorchitis. In contrast to animals, abortion is not a feature of brucellosis in pregnant women. Hypersensitivity reactions, which may mimic the symptoms of an infection, may occur in individuals who are exposed to infective material after previous, even subclinical, infection.

Structure

Brucellae are:

- Gram-negative coccobacilli (short rods) measuring about 0.6 to 1.5 μm by 0.5-0.7 μm.
- They are non-sporing and lack capsules or flagella and, therefore, are non-motile.
- The outer cell membrane closely resembles that of other Gram-negative bacilli with a dominant lipopolysaccharide (LPS) component and three main groups of proteins.
- The guanine-plus-cytosine content of the DNA is 55-58 moles/cm.
- No Brucella species has been found to harbour plasmids naturally although they readily accept broad-host-range plasmids.

- The metabolism of the brucellae is mainly oxidative and they show little action on carbohydrates in conventional media.
- They are aerobes but some species require an atmosphere with added CO_2 (5-10 per cent).
- Multiplication is slow at the optimum temperature of 37°C and enriched medium is needed to support adequate growth.

Brucella colonies become visible on suitable solid media in 2-3 days. The colonies of smooth strains are small, round and convex but dissociation, with loss of the O chains of the LPS, occurs readily to form rough or mucoid variants. These latter forms are natural in B canis and B ovis as the LPS of these lack O chains.

Classification and Antigenic Types

Distinguishing features of the six species of Brucella and their preferred hosts. B abortus, B melitensis and B suis are serious pathogens in humans, B canis causes mild disease and the other two species have not affected humans. A culture can be identified as belonging to the genus Brucella on the basis of colonial morphology, staining and slide agglutination with anti-Brucella serum, smooth or rough. Further classification is best done in a specialized laboratory.

Identification to species level may be done by the procedures. Further differentiation to biovars may be useful and is illustrated. As a further refinement, tests for the oxidative metabolism of certain aminoacids and carbohydrates have been devised. Modern DNA hybridization tests, however, show that the currently named species show a high degree of homology and suggest that the genus could be appropriately reclassified as having a single species.

- The application of techniques of molecular biology have allowed the cloning and characterization of several genes coding for outer membrane proteins,
- The use of PCR to identify the presence of brucellar DNA at genus and species level and the demonstration of species specific patterns of restriction fragment length polymorphism. It is predictable that this work will be extended to improve diagnostic tests and even vaccine development.

Two different O chains in brucellae occur in the LPS of the brucellae with smooth colonies. These are called A and M, nominally indicating abortus and melitensis antigens. ('Nominally', because some abortus biovars carry the M antigen and some common melitensis biovars the A antigen.) Both O chains have been shown to be homopolymers of 4,6-dideoxy-4-formamido-d-mannopyranose; they differ only in that in the A chain the sugar molecules are always linked 2-1 whereas the M chain has every fifth junction a 3-1 linkage. In routine serology, smooth species of brucellae cross-react almost completely with each other, but not with rough species and vice versa. Monospecific polyclonal sera reacting only to A or M antigens are prepared by cross absorption and monoclonal antibodies specific for A and M antigens are now available, indicating that there is at least one unique epitope on each type of chain.

CLASSIFICATIO OF BACTERIOLOGY

Bacteria are classified and identified to distinguish one organism from another and to group similar organisms by criteria of interest to microbiologists or other scientists. The most important level of this type of classification is the species level. A species name should mean the same thing to everyone. Within one species, strains and subgroups can differ by the disease they produce, their environmental habitat, and many other characteristics.

Formerly, species were created on the basis of such criteria, which may be extremely important for clinical microbiologists and physicians but which are not a sufficient basis for establishing a species. Verification of existing species and creation of new species should involve biochemical and other phenotypic criteria as well as DNA relatedness. In numerical or phenetic approaches to classification, strains are grouped on the basis of a large number of phenotypic characteristics. DNA relatedness is used to group strains on the basis of overall genetic similarity.

Species are identified in the clinical laboratory by morphological traits and biochemical tests, some of which are supplemented by serologic assessments (*e.g.*, identification of *Salmonella* and *Shigella* species). Because of differences in pathogenicity (*Escherichia coli*) or the necessity to characterize a disease outbreak (*Vibrio cholerae*, methicillin-resistant *Staphylococcus aureus*), strains of medical interest are often classified below the species level by serology or identification of toxins. Pathogenic or epidemic strains also can be classified by the presence of a specific plasmid, by their plasmid profile (the number and sizes of plasmids), or by bacteriophage susceptibility patterns (phage typing). Newer molecular biologic techniques have enabled scientists to identify some species and strains (without the use of biochemical tests) by identifying a specific gene or genetic sequence, sometimes directly from the clinical specimen.

Laboratories have no difficulty in identifying typical strains of common bacteria using commonly available test systems. Problems do arise, however, when atypical strains or rare or newly described species are not in the data base. Such difficulties are compounded when the strains are misidentified rather than unidentified, and so laboratory personnel and physicians (at least infectious diseases specialists) should be familiar with taxonomic reference texts and journals that publish papers on new species. Bacterial nomenclature at the genus and species level changes often, based primarily on the use of newer genetic techniques. A species may acquire more than one name. In some cases the recognition of a new species results in a unique correlation with specific clinical problems. For example, recognition of *Porphyromonas gingivalis* as a unique species, separate from its previous inclusion within *Bacteroides melaninogenicus* (now known to be composed of several taxonomic groups of black-pigmenting anaerobic gram-negative bacilli), elucidated its role as a key pathogen in adult periodontitis. It is important to understand why these changes and synonyms exist in taxonomy.

The clinical laboratory is concerned with the rapid, sensitive, and accurate identification of microbes involved in producing disease. The number and types of tests done in such a laboratory depend on its size and the population it serves. Highly specialized or rarely performed tests should be done only by reference laboratories. Physicians, clinical laboratory personnel, and reference laboratory personnel must have a good working relationship if patients are to receive first-rate care. In addition, the physician and the clinical laboratory personnel must know which diseases and isolates are reportable to public health laboratories and how to report them.

Definitions of Bacteriology

Taxonomy

Taxonomy is the science of classification, identification, and nomenclature. For classification purposes, organisms are usually organized into subspecies, species, genera, families, and higher orders. For eukaryotes, the definition of the species usually stresses the ability of similar organisms to reproduce sexually with the formation of a zygote and to produce fertile offspring. However, bacteria do not undergo sexual reproduction in the eukaryotic sense. Other criteria are used for their classification.

Classification

Classification is the orderly arrangement of bacteria into groups. There is nothing inherently scientific about classification, and different groups of scientists may classify the same organisms differently.

For example, clinical microbiologists are interested in the serotype, antimicrobial resistance pattern, and toxin and invasiveness factors in *Escherichia coli*, whereas geneticists are concerned with specific mutations and plasmids.

Identification

Identification is the practical use of classification criteria to distinguish certain organisms from others, to verify the authenticity or utility of a strain or a particular reaction, or to isolate and identify the organism that causes a disease.

Nomenclature

Nomenclature (naming) is the means by which the characteristics of a species are defined and communicated among microbiologists.

A species name should mean the same thing to all microbiologists, yet some definitions vary in different countries or microbiologic specialty groups. For example, the organism known as *Clostridium perfringens* in the United States is called*Clostridium welchii* in England.

Species

A bacterial species is a distinct organism with certain characteristic features, or a group of organisms that resemble one another closely in the most important features of their organization.

In the past, unfortunately, there was little agreement about these criteria or about the number of features necessary to distinguish a species. Species were often defined solely by such criteria as host range, pathogenicity, or ability to produce gas during the fermentation of a given sugar.

Without a universal consensus, criteria reflected the interests of the investigators who described a particular species. For example, bacteria that caused plant diseases were often defined by the plant from which they were isolated; also, each new *Salmonella* serotype that was discovered was given species status.

These practices have been replaced by generally accepted genetic criteria that can be used to define species in all groups of bacteria.

Approaches to Taxonomy

Numerical Approach

In their studies on members of the family Enterobacteriaceae, Edwards and Ewing established the following principles to characterize, classify, and identify organisms (Lennette *et al.*, 1985): Classification and identification of an organism should be based on its overall morphologic and biochemical pattern. A single characteristic (pathogenicity, host range, or biochemical reaction), regardless of its importance, is not a sufficient basis for classifying or identifying an organism. A large and diverse strain sample must be tested to determine accurately the biochemical characteristics used to distinguish a given species. Atypical strains often are perfectly typical members of a given biogroup within an existing species, but sometimes they are typical members of an unrecognized new species.

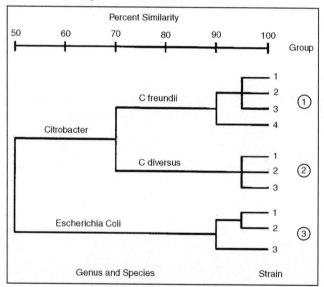

Fig. Example of Dendrogramw

In numerical taxonomy (also called computer or phenetic taxonomy) many (50 to 200) biochemical, morphological, and cultural characteristics, as well as susceptibilities to antibiotics and inorganic compounds, are used to determine the degree of similarity between organisms. In numerical studies, investigators often calculate the coefficient of similarity or percentage of similarity between strains (where strain indicates a single isolate from a specimen). A dendrogram or a similarity matrix is constructed that joins individual strains into groups and places one group with other groups on the basis of their percentage of similarity. The group 1 represents three *Citrobacter freundii* strains that are about 95 per cent similar and join with a fourth *C. freundii* strain at the level of 90 per cent similarity. Group 2 is composed of three *Citrobacter diversus* strains that are 95 per cent similar, and group 3 contains two *E. coli* strains that are 95 per cent similar, as well as a third *E. coli* strain to which they are 90 per cent similar. Similarity between groups 1 and 2 occurs at the 70 per cent level, and group 3 is about 50 per cent similar to groups 1 and 2.

In some cases, certain characteristics may be weighted more heavily; for example, the presence of spores in *Clostridium* might be weighted more heavily than the organism's ability to use a specific carbon source. A given level of similarity can be equated with relatedness at the genus, species, and, sometimes, subspecies levels. For instance, strains of a given species may cluster at a 90 per cent similarity level, species within a given genus may cluster at the 70 per cent level, and different genera in the same family may cluster at the 50 per cent or lower level.

When this approach is the only basis for defining a species, it is difficult to know how many and which tests should be chosen; whether and how the tests should be weighted; and what level of similarity should be chosen to reflect relatedness at the genus and species levels. Most bacteria have enough DNA to specify some 1,500 to 6,000 average-sized genes. Therefore, even a battery of 300 tests would assay only 5 to 20 per cent of the genetic potential of a bacterium.

Tests that are comparatively simple to conduct (such as those for carbohydrate utilization and for enzymes, presence of which can be assayed colourimetrically) are performed more often than tests for structural, reproductive, and regulatory genes, presence of which is difficult to assay. Thus, major differences may go undetected. Other types of errors may occur when species are classified solely on the basis of phenotype. For example, different enzymes (specified by different genes) may catalyze the same reaction. Also, even if a metabolic gene is functional, negative reactions can occur because of the inability of the substrate to enter the cell, because of a mutation in a regulatory gene, or by production of an inactive protein. There is not necessarily a one-to-one correlation between a reaction and the number of genes needed to carry out that reaction.

For instance, six enzymatic steps may be involved in a given pathway. If an assay for the end product is performed, a positive reaction indicates the presence of all six enzymes, whereas a negative reaction can mean the absence or non-function of one to six enzymes. Several other strain characteristics can affect phenotypic characterization; these include growth rate, incubation temperature, salt requirement, and pH. Plasmids that carry metabolic genes can enable strains to carry out reactions atypical for strains of that species. The same set of "definitive" reactions cannot be used to classify all groups of organisms, and there is no standard number of specific reactions that allows identification of a species. Organisms are identified on the basis of phenotype, but, from the taxonomic standpoint, definition of species solely on this basis is subject to error.

Phylogenetic Approach

The ideal means of identifying and classifying bacteria would be to compare each gene sequence in a given strain with the gene sequences for every known species.

This cannot be done, but the total DNA of one organism can be compared with that of any other organism by a method called nucleic acid hybridization or DNA hybridization. This method can be used to measure the number of DNA sequences that any two organisms have in common and to estimate the percentage of divergence within DNA sequences that are related but not identical. DNA relatedness studies have been done for yeasts, viruses, bacteriophages, and many groups of bacteria.

Five factors can be used to determine DNA relatedness: genome size, guanine-plus-cytosine (G+C) content, DNA relatedness under conditions optimal for DNA reassociation, thermal stability of related DNA sequences, and DNA relatedness under conditions supraoptimal for DNA reassociation. Because it is not practical to conduct these genotypic or phylogenetic evaluations in clinical laboratories, the results of simpler tests usually must be correlated with known phylogenetic data. For example, yellow strains of*Enterobacter cloacae* were shown, by DNA relatedness, to form a separate species, *Enterobacter sakazakii*, but were not designated as such until results of practical tests were correlated with the DNA data to allow routine laboratories to identify the new species.

Genome Size

True bacterial DNAs have genome sizes (measured as molecular weight) between 1×10^9 and 8×10^9. Genome size determinations sometimes can distinguish between groups. They were used to distinguish *Legionella pneumophila* (the legionnaire's disease bacterium) from *Bartonella (Rickettsia) quintana*, the agent of trench fever. *L. pneumophila* has a genome size of about 3×10^9; that of *B. quintana* is about 1×10^9.

Guanine-plus-Cytosine Content

The G+C content in bacterial DNA ranges from about 25 to 75 per cent. This percentage is specific, but not exclusive, for a species; two strains with a similar G+C content may or may not belong to the same species. If the G+C contents are very different, however, the strains cannot be members of the same species.

DNA Relatedness under Conditions Optimal for DNA Reassociation

DNA relatedness is determined by allowing single-stranded DNA from one strain to reassociate with single-stranded DNA from a second strain, to form a double-stranded DNA molecule. This is a specific, temperature-dependent reaction. The optimal temperature for DNA reassociation is 25 to 30°C below the temperature at which native double-stranded DNA denatures into single strands. Many studies indicate that a bacterial species is composed of strains that are 70 to 100 per cent related. In contrast, relatedness between different species is 0 to about 65 per cent. It is important to emphasize that the term "related" does not mean "identical" or "homologous." Similar but non-identical nucleic acid sequences can reassociate.

Thermal Stability of Related DNA Sequences

Each 1 per cent of unpaired nucleotide bases in a double-stranded DNA sequence causes a 1 per cent decrease in the thermal stability of that DNA duplex. Therefore, a comparison between the thermal stability of a control double-stranded molecule (in which both strands of DNA are from the same organism) and that of a heteroduplex (DNA strands from two different organisms) allows assessment of divergence between related nucleotide sequences.

DNA Relatedness under Supraoptimal Conditions for DNA Reassociation

When the incubation temperature used for DNA reassociation is raised from 25-30° C below the denaturation temperature to only 10-15° C below the denaturation temperature, only very closely related (and therefore highly thermally stable) DNA sequences can reassociate. Strains from the same species are 60 per cent or more related at these supraoptimal incubation temperatures.

Defining Species on the Basis of DNA Relatedness

Use of these five factors allows a species definition based on DNA. Thus, *E. coli* can be defined as a series of strains with a G+C content of 49 to 52 moles per cent, a genome molecular weight of 2.3×10^9 to 3.0×10^9, relatedness of 70 per cent or more at an optimal reassociation temperature with 0 to 4 per cent divergence in related sequences, and relatedness of 60 per cent or more at a supraoptimal reassociation temperature.

Experience with more than 300 species has produced an arbitrary phylogenetic definition of a species to which most taxonomists subscribe: "strains with approximately 70 per cent or greater DNA-DNA relatedness and with 5° C or less divergence in related sequences."

When these two criteria are met, genome size and G+C content are always similar, and relatedness is almost always 60 per cent or more at supraoptimal incubation temperatures. The 70 per cent species relatedness rule has been ignored occasionally when the existing nomenclature is deeply ingrained, as is that for *E. coli* and the four *Shigella* species.

Because these organisms are all 70 per cent or more related, DNA studies indicate that they should be grouped into a single species, instead of the present five species in two genera.

This change has not been made because of the presumed confusion that would result. DNA relatedness provides one species definition that can be applied equally to all organisms. Moreover, it cannot be affected by phenotypic variation, mutations, or the presence or absence of metabolic or other plasmids. It measures overall relatedness, and these factors affect only a very small percentage of the total DNA.

Polyphasic Approach

In practice, the approach to bacterial taxonomy should be polyphasic. The first step is phenotypic grouping of strains by morphological, biochemical and any other characteristics of interest. The phenotypic groups are then tested for DNA relatedness to determine whether the observed phenotypic homogeneity (or heterogeneity) is reflected by phylogenetic homogeneity or heterogeneity. The third and most important step is reexamination of the biochemical characteristics of the DNA relatedness groups.

This allows determination of the biochemical borders of each group and determination of reactions of diagnostic value for the group. For identification of a given organism, the importance of specific tests is weighted on the basis of correlation with DNA results. Occasionally, the reactions commonly used will not distinguish completely between two distinct DNA relatedness groups. In these cases, other biochemical tests of diagnostic value must be sought.

CONTROL OF BRUCELLA MELITENSIS

Natural and preferred animal hosts

Goats are classically the natural hosts of *Brucella melitensis* while sheep are the preferred hosts. This definition relates to the fact that *B. melitensis* preferably causes abortion in the goats, but infected sheep will as well abort. The abortion usually occurs as a single event, in the last trimester of gestation that follows the infection. Since the aborted placenta and fetus are massively contaminated with *Brucella* they lead to the dissemination of the organisms in the environment and to exposure of uninfected animals to the disease. Migrating flocks, therefore, present a major risk to dairy cattle herds and to intensively managed flocks that are fed on fodder harvested from these fields. Another possible route of infection may occur through direct contact with infected flocks when common pasture is used. Canides and other carnivores present special risk to intensively managed livestock (and their human owners) as they scavenge and may carry the aborted material to clean areas.

B. melitensis is the most virulent species of all the brucellae (2). The virulence is partly measured by their capacity to cause brucellosis in cattle and human beings that are not considered natural or preferred hosts (3), even though in these species the disease may sporadically lead to abortion. Moreover, *B. melitensis* is excreted in the milk of infected cows thus transmitting the disease to the suckling neo-natals. The fact that brucellosis can revert to latency would suggest that a certain amount of animals could be silent carriers of the disease. Many of the gestating dams can, therefore, transfer the disease in utero to the fetuses or post natally to the offspring throughout lactation. It is therefore recommended to remove both the infected dams and their offspring when conducting eradication programmes in infected flocks or herds.

B. melitensis causes epididymis and orchitis in the males. This can present another source of infection, or mode of transmission, in flocks where natural mating is practiced. Especially, the exchange of males amongst breeders of extensively managed flocks in endemic areas can similarly lead to dissemination of the disease by the infected males. Control programmes need to address this issue mainly by restricting the animal movement.

The sharing amongst breeders of common grazing pastures lends to intermingling of infected flocks with brucellosis clean flocks. The uninfected animals will therefore be exposed to the disease from multiple sources such as abortion discharges; direct contact and airborne particles. Despite the lack of solid evidence we believe that the latest route has been so far underestimated as one of the important factors that affect the dissemination of *Brucella* in the field. This conclusion was reached when we identified infection of intensively managed dairy cattle herds with *B. melitensis*. Epidemiological examination of the cases has clearly demonstrated the lack of direct contact between the infected cattle and the sheep flocks that surrounded the holdings, neither could it be confirmed that the cows were fed with contaminated fodder. Since no other sources could be identified, it was speculated that the disease was transmitted to the cows by an air borne route. The fact, however, that the infected cattle did not usually abort due to *B. melitensis* did not reduce the spread of the disease amongst the cows.

The mechanisms by which *Brucella* was disseminated in these holdings was not clear. We may assume that similar principles that govern the spread of *B. melitensis* amongst sheep and goats also applied to the cow population. In dairy herds, however, additional means could be considered. As *Brucella* organisms were excreted in the milk it was very likely that the repeated milking using the same automatic cups, twice or three times a day, may have led to mechanical transfer of the organisms from cow to cow. Milk dripping from the teats could also increase the contamination of the environment lending to aerosols that could be absorbed through the epithelial linings of the conjunctiva and the respiratory tracts.

B. melitensis is not associated with abortion storms in cattle. Clinically evident abortions that usually attract the attention of the attending veterinarians to a possible infection do not generally occur. It is, therefore, necessary in endemic areas to develop alternative monitoring approaches in order to facilitate identification of *B. melitensis* infected herds. In a recent brucella outbreak, however, cows infected with *B. melitensis* aborted at the onset of the infection in the herd. We confirmed the involvement of the brucellae in the abortion by direct isolation of the strain from the aborted placentas and fetuses. The dams had seroconverted either prior to, or immediately after the abortion. It was debatable, therefore, whether it was genetic susceptiblity that led these cows to abort or whether it was due to evolutionary changes in *B. melitensis* that endowed the organisms with the abortive capacity in cows?

The eradication of *B. melitensis* from dairy cattle involve additional concerns in comparison to the eradication of *B. abortus*. Humans easily contract *B. melitensis* due to the extremely low inoculum dose required to establish infection. Since the bacteria are excreted in the milk, which in the cow is produced in large quantities, the requirement to remove the udder and internal organs from slaughtered cows would necessarily lead to exposure of the abattoir personnel to huge amounts of the organisms. To reduce the risks it is therefore recommended that the cows be dried off prior to sending them to slaughter.

Serodiagnosis

The implementation of an effective surveillance programme is a prerequisit to the successful control of *B. melitensis*. The method which will best serve the programme also depends on whether the animals were vaccinated, on the basic infrastructure of the veterinary services regarding the availability of advanced equipment and skilled personnel, and necessitates as a prerequisit a commitment to destroy the infected animals, whether for compensation or voluntarily.

The Rev.1 is a live vaccine strain (4), bearing similar smooth SLPS antigens that are utilized in most serological methods. Vaccination of the animals, therefore, lends to development of antibodies that are normally elicited by infection, thus interfering with surveillance programmes. Several approaches have been developed to overcome this problem. The common approach is to only vaccinate the ewe-lambs and kid goats between the ages of 2 to 6 months and exclude them from the serological tests until their vaccine titers disappear. Since, however, depending on the serological method different antibody isotypes are revealed it is suggested that the animals be tested only after their first parturation which is more than half a year after their date of vaccination. In this case only a minor portion of the population will react in the complement fixation test (CFT) and the Rose Bengal test (RBT).

Another approach would be to test the sera by competitive ELISA, a recently developed technique that distinguishes between seropositive reactors due to vaccination or infection. This technique has been confirmed to be both specific and sensitive and its use is fairly simple (8). Even though in principle the method allows the diagnosis of different target hosts, it has been only standardized for cattle. This method is applicable in countries that have access to mass supply of the reagents at low costs, and is using software controlled automated equipment. The concern of distinguishing between vaccinated animals as opposed to infected ones has recently received an additional breakthrough.

A new vaccine, based on live attenuated *B. abortus* RB51 strain, has been shown to confer excellent protection to the cattle. This strain is deficient in the smooth O-chain antigen that characterizes the normal strains. As a result, vaccination with this strain does not elicit anti smooth O-chain antibodies thus eliminating the problem of distinguishing between vaccinated and infected animals. In contrast, infection with the normal strain will develop anti-smooth antibodies that are identified by the serodiagnostic tests. In the event that animals are not vaccinated the problem of distinguishing between vaccination and infection does not apply.

On the other hand, where vaccination is not practiced, the flocks remain susceptible to the disease and besides abortion there is no indication of the onset of the disease. As a result, flocks should be routinely surveyed using highly sensitive and specific methods, however, at low costs. The Rose Bengal Test (RBT) is precisely such a method that fits these criteria. It is a simple screening method that reveals positive reactors at sensitivity and specificity almost equivalent to CFT.

Neither skilled personnel nor advanced equipment are required to perform the test and it can, therefore, be conducted in peripheral laboratories. The major drawback of this test is the reduced sensitivity that has been shown to occur with O-chain M-bearing *Brucella* strains (12). This is due to the fact that the antigen used in the test bears O-chain A antigen (*B. abortus* strain 1119). One should also bear in mind that because the disease can present in different livestock in complicated phases, and because different management systems are applied in the rearing of the flocks, none of the serological tests alone can identify all positive reactors.

It is recommended, therefore, that more than one diagnostic method be applied throughout the implementation of a surveillance programme.

The most complicated problems are encountered in countries where although vaccination is applied the coverage is only partial. Thus, mixed populations of vaccinated and infected animals might constitute a single flock. In this case, it is recommended to use CFT as the leading confirmative diagnostic method.

Alternatively, c-ELISA may be used as a screening method (to directly exclude positive reactors due to vaccination) while i-ELISA should be used as a confirmatory test. The use of ELISA has the drawback that it does not give end point titers making the judgement of the results obtained from suspected reactors more difficult. The CFT has the advantage over the ELISA methods also because A antigen and M antigen can be used simultaneously thereby increasing the probability that positive reactors will not be missed. This issue is critical when testing cattle in areas that are endemic with *B. melitensis*.

Bacteriological Diagnosis

Knowing the epidemiology is a key element of a successful control programme. The gold standard that confirms the disease is the isolation of the bacterial agent. Subsequently the strain should be biotyped to identify its species and biovar. The identification of the cause of the disease is important since none of the *Brucella* species is as hazardous to the human population as *B. melitensis*. Moreover, export/import trade agreements amongst countries require that only brucellosis free animals be transferred in order to exclude the possible importation of a new *Brucella* species to the country. On the local level, the existence of different *Brucella* biotypes amongst the *Brucella* species facilitated the identification of the source of the infection (13). This is extremely important in areas that have mixed populations of sheep, goats and cattle since *B. melitensis* is easily introduced into the cattle population.

The problem of *B. melitensis* in cattle requires further consideration. Firstly, dairy cattle usually constitutes the reservoir for the national milk industry leading to dissemination of contaminated milk to the whole population. Secondly, different control approaches are required for *B. abortus* and *B. melitensis* infections. *B. abortus* is the causative agent of abortion in cattle thereby leading to epizootic spread of the disease amongst the cows. In contrast, *B. melitensis* does not usually cause abortion in cattle which therefore tend to reduce the disemination of the disease in the herd due to containment of the organisms in the infected animals. *B. melitensis* will usually spread within the herd only if it remains undetected. Thirdly, if a test and slaughter eradication programme is applied the cows infeceted with *B. melitensis* pose a threat to the abattoir personnel who are exposed to huge amounts of the organisms during slaughter. Spillage of the milk from the udder when removed from the carcass for destruction presents the major risk to abattoir personnel and has been documented to lead to human infection. It is therefore recommended that dairy cows be dried off prior to slaughter.

A special concern should be given to countries using a live vaccine strain. Adverse effects of persistent survival and excretion of the bacteria in the milk have been confirmed amongst cattle, and sheep and goats, that were vaccinated with live *B. abortus* S19 and *B. melitensis* Rev.1 vaccines, respectively (14-19). Herds and flocks that have been shown to include excretors of the vaccine strain should not be considered infected. Nevertheless, the excreting animals should be destroyed to prevent further exposure of additional animals to the strain. This information can only be obtained if direct isolation of the infective agent is attempted and followed by biotyping of the isolated strain. In a recent field study a mixed infection of a flock with Rev.1 vaccine strain and a field strain had been diagnosed. In one case, a mixed infection was observed in an aborting ewe-lamb that received Rev.1 vaccine few months earlier. In other cases horizontal transfer of the vaccine strain was demonstrated either as a smooth strain or as a rough isolate. These results raised a debate on the safety.

The biotyping of *Brucella* isolates can be performed by conventional bacteriological techniques. Recently, *omp2* gene sequence based PCR techniques have been established as additional diagnostic methods and some relying on the *omp2* gene sequences being used as *Brucella* spp. biotyping methods. The technique is advantageous over conventional biotyping methods, providing faster results and facilitating the testing of samples from suspect materials (contaminated aborted placenta, lymph nodes, semen, blood). The reduced sensitivity, mostly revealing not less than 10 microorganisms, is a major drawback. Moreover, since an isolate is not obtained unknown characteristics will remain vague and it will be impossible to obtain epidemiological data on the source of the infection or whether new phenotypes/genotypes develop.

Prophylaxis

Brucellosis has been known for over a century. Throughout the years the scientific community has gained solid information on the disease and its prophylaxis. It has been demonstrated that vaccination is the best prophylactic means to protect the environment. Firstly, it confers good protection against abortions as well as to other *Brucella* shedding mechanisms - *e.g.*, secretion of the strain in the milk. Secondly, vaccination confers humoral and cellular immune protection that can limit horizontal transfer of the organisms. Only a few vaccines have been widely accepted as good candidates for brucellosis prophylaxis. Among these, the original *B. melitensis* Elberg strain has recently been proposed as a superior vaccine, compared to *B. abortus* S19 and *B. suis* S2. It has ben shown that the Rev. 1 vaccine not only protects against *B. melitensis* but it also protects other animal species against *B. abortus* or *B. suis*. Inspite of this information the traditional approach is still dominant, suggesting that the homologous vaccine species - *e.g.*, *B. abortus*, *B. melitensis*, and *B. suis*, be applied against each disease, respectively.

B. abortus S19 is the most popular vaccine against *B. abortus*. It had been widely used as a subcutaneous, full dose inoculum. Female calves were considered the target population in order to reduce the adverse effects of the vaccine when adult animal population was vaccinated. These effects were mostly humoral and rarely strain persistence occurred in the vaccinated animals. The control of the disease, however, requires that test and slaughter be carried out simultaneously with the vaccination programme. This lends to enormous expenses due to the compensation paid for the destruction of the infected animals. Several practitioners have suggested that such a programme is too expensive for most countries and rather than facilitating the eradication it will slow it because of budget limits. As a result new approaches have been sought to overcome this obstacle.

Two new approaches have been tested. The first approach implemented an ocular route for vaccination, using a reduced dose. This method allowed vaccination of adult animals even during pregnancy without causing abortion or persistent serological responses. It was therefore possible to repeat the vaccination in endemic populations without the need for slaughter compensation of the infected herds. The second approach applied a rough vaccine strain. It was suggested that the rough form would not elicit anti smooth O-chain antigen, the predominant antigen of the normal strain, thus allowing its use as a vaccine. It was simultaneously expected that the mutation from smooth to rough would attenuate the strain to sufficiently reduce its virulence. As a result vaccination with the rough strain has been suggested to prevent adverse humoral responses that hamper surveillance programmes.

The RB51 is a recent vaccine strain that was developed according to these principles. This vaccine is inoculated subcutaneously, and can be applied in adult animals without causing abortion. Since anti smooth O-chain antibodies are not elicited, it is possible to repeat vaccination without hampering surveillance programmes. It is therefore considered an improved alternative to the S19 vaccine. Nevertheless, the implementation of use of this vaccine in practice has been limited. It has only recently been tested on a pilot scale and approved by the USDA for commercial use. Still unknown are the side effects and efficacy of use of this vaccine in small ruminants.

The small ruminant's equivalent vaccine as is *B. abortus* S19 in cattle. Since 1957, when first used in international pilot scale studies, this vaccine had been used worldwide showing excellent results in the control of *B. melitensis*. Because of its wide use different producers became interested in mass production of the vaccine for commercial purposes. The seed stock had then been distributed among the producers, each propagating it similarly, however, losing to a certain extent the quality of the vaccine. As a result some countries have encountered adverse effects with the vaccine, the most controversial being South Africa where a vaccine revertant caused animal and human brucellosis. A similar, but less severe infection has been observed in Israel.

These results led to questioning the application of the vaccine in a regional control programme for the Middle East countries, proposed by the FAO/WHO/OIE expert committee. The programme included a decision to vaccinate the small ruminant population with a reduced dose, every two years, for a period of ten years. Only after reducing the infection rates amongst the flocks could the countries begin a second stage of a test and slaughter scheme. It was argued that since the vaccine strain had lost important immunogenic properties, such a programme would hamper surveillance without achieving effective control. This debate led to the assembling of the *Brucella* experts aimed at the evaluation. The following conclusions were drawn: Firstly, it was noted that the original Elberg, the only seed stock permitted for use, has been deposited in the European Pharmacopoeia. Secondly, it was suggested that production of the vaccine should conform to the methods described in the OIE manual of Standards for Diagnostic Tests and Vaccines (2). Thirdly, it was recommended that the regional project should include bacteriological monitoring to obtain a clear epidemiological figure of the existence of the disease in the area. Lastly, a call for developing serological methods that will distinguish between infected and vaccinated animals has been made. The ocular vaccination with a reduced dose of 10^8 c.f.u. has been suggested as one of the solutions.

These recommendations were endorsed for the second time in a WHO expert meeting on development/improvement of *Brucella* vaccines. The unanimously accepted as the recommended vaccine to obtain effective control of the disease. The Rev.1 vaccine has been also considered a significant alternative to the S19 vaccine for the protection of cattle, provided that sufficient evidence is gained from controlled cow vaccination experiments. The use of the *B. suis* S2 as a vaccine has been evaluated in two major aspects. Firstly, since first introduced in China the vaccine had been used in this country in large scales.

The concept at the beginning was to use oral vaccination by seeding the drinking water with the vaccine. This concept had later been withdrawn as it was difficult to confirm the dose of the vaccine administered to any animal. The direct oral inoculation of the vaccine was, therefore, preferred. According to the Chinese authorities, the S2 vaccination gained success lending to continuation of this programme despite the recommendations made on the use of the Rev.1 vaccine. As far as China was concerned the S2 vaccine was preferable due to its capacity to protect all important domestic farm animals - *e.g.*, small ruminants, cattle and swine. Moreover, the dispensing of the vaccine in the drinking water allowed mass vaccination of the huge animal population that was otherwise inaccessible to the practitioners. The second approach was to test the efficacy of the vaccine in controlled laboratory experiments.

Multi-disciplinary Collaboration among the Laboratory

A multi-disciplinary collaboration among the laboratory, the veterinary field services and the public health services is imperative to the implementation of a successful control programme. The laboratory provides the expertise in diagnosis, the veterinary services are in charge of the eradication programme and the public health services are expected to diagnose the human population and treat infected patients. Brucellosis has been designated a notifiable disease. The soverignty of the veterinary services and the public health services lends to independent diagnosis of the disease among the animal and the human populations, respectively. This can be advantageous in the sense that a double surveillance system is applied in the diagnosis of the disease. The occurrence of the infection in the livestock is notified to the public health services to increase the physicians' awareness to the possible existence of the disease in the human population. Similarly, when the physicians identify infected persons they should notify the veterinary services to initiate surveillance of the livestock to track the infection source. The main drawback in this approach however is that it leads to the development of different monitoring approaches thereby disrupting harmonization. The diagnostic laboratory thus acts as a link between the two organizations by playing an instrumental role in coordination and standardization of the methods. Moreover, the reference laboratory provides expertise in *Brucella* biotyping from human and animal sources.

The harmonization of the control programme can better be achieved by establishing a national steering committee. Members of the committee should include veterinarians, physicians and laboratory personnel. The participation of administrators from the public health services is recommended. This committee should outline the principles that will dictate the activities of the three participating components.

The committe should make an elementary decision as to whether or not the veterinary services will instigate vaccination. Similarly, it should decide upon the surveillance scheme and the criteria used to judge the results. Specifically, depending on the diagnostic method, cut off values should be determined that will distinguish between positive, suspected and negative reactors.

These criteria will establish the basis for compensation when slaughtering the infected animals. In addition, the committee should ensure that replacement stocks be established and, if possible, to characterize the conditions that will allow approval of a brucellosis free status to designated intensively managed farms. Finally, the committee should organize an education campaign targeted at the breeders and their families and at the rural and urban populations.

PHENOTYPIC CHARACTERISTICS USEFUL IN CLASSIFICATION AND IDENTIFICATION

Morphologic Characteristics

Both wet-mounted and properly stained bacterial cell suspensions can yield a great deal of information. These simple tests can indicate the Gram reaction of the organism; whether it is acid-fast; its motility; the arrangement of its flagella; the presence of spores, capsules, and inclusion bodies; and, of course, its shape.

This information often can allow identification of an organism to the genus level, or can minimize the possibility that it belongs to one or another group. Colony characteristics and pigmentation are also quite helpful. For example, colonies of several *Porphyromonas* species autofluoresce under long-wavelength ultraviolet light, and *Proteus* species swarm on appropriate media.

Growth Characteristics

A primary distinguishing characteristic is whether an organism grows aerobically, anaerobically, facultatively (*i.e.*, in either the presence or absence of oxygen), or microaerobically (*i.e.*, in the presence of a less than atmospheric partial pressure of oxygen). The proper atmospheric conditions are essential for isolating and identifying bacteria. Other important growth assessments include the incubation temperature, pH, nutrients required, and resistance to antibiotics. For example, one diarrheal disease agent,*Campylobacter jejuni*, grows well at 42° C in the presence of several antibiotics; another, *Y. enterocolitica*, grows better than most other bacteria at 4° C. *Legionella, Haemophilus*, and some other pathogens require specific growth factors, whereas *E. coli* and most other Enterobacteriaceae can grow on minimal media.

Antigens and Phage Susceptibility

Cell wall (O), flagellar (H), and capsular (K) antigens are used to aid in classifying certain organisms at the species level, to serotype strains of medically important species for epidemiologic purposes, or to identify serotypes of public health importance. Serotyping is also sometimes used to distinguish strains of exceptional virulence or public health importance, for example with *V. cholerae* (O1 is the pandemic strain) and *E. coli* (enterotoxigenic, enteroinvasive, enterohemorrhagic, and enteropathogenic serotypes).

Phage typing (determining the susceptibility pattern of an isolate to a set of specific bacteriophages) has been used primarily as an aid in epidemiologic surveillance of diseases caused by *Staphylococcus aureus*, mycobacteria, *P, aeruginosa*, *V. cholerae*, and *S. typhi*. Susceptibility to bacteriocins has also been used as an epidemiologic strain marker. In most cases recently, phage and bacteriocin typing have been supplanted by molecular methods.

Biochemical Characteristics

Most bacteria are identified and classified largely on the basis of their reactions in a series of biochemical tests.

Some tests are used routinely for many groups of bacteria (oxidase, nitrate reduction, amino acid degrading enzymes, fermentation or utilization of carbohydrates); others are restricted to a single family, genus, or species (coagulase test for staphylococci, pyrrolidonyl arylamidase test for Gram-positive cocci).

Both the number of tests needed and the actual tests used for identification vary from one group of organisms to another. Therefore, the lengths to which a laboratory should go in detecting and identifying organisms must be decided in each laboratory on the basis of its function, the type of population it serves, and its resources.

Clinical laboratories today base the extent of their work on the clinical relevance of an isolate to the particular patient from which it originated, the public health significance of complete identification, and the overall cost-benefit analysis of their procedures. For example, the Centers for Disease Control and Prevention (CDC) reference laboratory uses at least 46 tests to identify members of the Enterobacteriaceae, whereas most clinical laboratories, using commercial identification kits or simple rapid tests, identify isolates with far fewer criteria.

Classification Below and Above the Species Level

Below the Species Level

Particularly for epidemiological purposes, clinical microbiologists must distinguish strains with particular traits from other strains in the same species. For example, serotype O157:H7 *E. coli* are identified in stool specimens because of their association with bloody diarrhea and subsequent hemolytic uremic syndrome.

Below the species level, strains are designated as groups or types on the basis of common serologic or biochemical reactions, phage or bacteriocin sensitivity, pathogenicity, or other characteristics. Many of these characteristics are already used and accepted: serotype, phage type, colicin type, biotype, bioserotype (a group of strains from the same species with common biochemical and serologic characteristics that set them apart from other members of the species), and pathotype (*e.g.*, toxigenic*Clostridium difficile*, invasive *E. coli*, and toxigenic *Corynebacterium diphtheriae*).

Above the Species Level

In addition to species and subspecies designations, clinical microbiologists must be familiar with genera and families. A genus is a group of related species, and a family is a group of related genera.

An ideal genus would be composed of species with similar phenotypic and phylogenetic characteristics. Some phenotypically homogeneous genera approach this criterion (*Citrobacter, Yersinia,* and *Serratia*). More often, however, the phenotypic similarity is present, but the genetic relatedness is not. *Bacillus, Clostridium,* and *Legionella* are examples of accepted phenotypic genera in which genetic relatedness between species is not 50 to 65 per cent, but 0 to 65 per cent. When phenotypic and genetic similarity are not both present, phenotypic similarity generally should be given priority in establishing genera. Identification practices are simplified by having the most phenotypically similar species in the same genus. The primary consideration for a genus is that it contain biochemically similar species that are convenient or important to consider as a group separate from other groups of organisms. The sequencing of ribosomal RNA (rRNA) genes, which have been highly conserved through evolution, allows phylogenetic comparisons to be made between species whose total DNAs are essentially unrelated. It also allows phylogenetic classification at the genus, family, and higher taxonomic levels. The rRNA sequence data are usually not used to designate genera or families unless supported by similarities in phenotypic tests.

Designation of New Species and Nomenclatural Changes

Species are named according to principles and rules of nomenclature set forth in the Bacteriological Code. Scientific names are taken from Latin or Greek. The correct name of a species or higher taxon is determined by three criteria: valid publication, legitimacy of the name with regard to the rules of nomenclature, and priority of publication (that is, it must be the first validly published name for the taxon).

To be published validly, a new species proposal must contain the species name, a description of the species, and the designation of a type strain for the species, and the name must be published in the *International Journal for Systematic Bacteriology (IJSB)*. Once proposed, a name does not go through a formal process to be accepted officially; in fact, the opposite is true—a validly published name is assumed to be correct unless and until it is challenged officially. A challenge is initiated by publishing a request for an opinion (to the Judicial Commission of the International Association of Microbiological Societies) in the *IJSB*.

This occurs only in cases in which the validity of a name is questioned with respect to compliance with the rules of the Bacteriological Code. A question of classification that is based on scientific data (for example, whether a species, on the basis of its biochemical or genetic characteristics, or both, should be placed in a new genus or an existing genus) is not settled by the Judicial Commission, but by the preference and usage of the scientific community. This is why there are pairs of names such as *Providencia rettgeri/ Proteus rettgeri*, *Moraxella catarrhalis/Branhamella catarrhalis*, and *Legionella micdadei/Tatlockia micdadei*. More than one name may thus exist for a single organism. This is not, however, restricted to bacterial nomenclature. Multiple names exist for many antibiotics and other drugs and enzymes.

A number of genera have been divided into additional genera and species have been moved to new or existing genera, such as *Arcobacter* (new genus for former members of *Campylobacter*) and *Burkholderia* species (formerly species of *Pseudomonas*). Two former *Campylobacter* species (*cinaedi* and *fennelliae*) have been moved to the existing genus *Helicobacter* in another example. The best source of information for new species proposals and nomenclatural changes is the *IJSB*. In addition, the *Journal of Clinical Microbiology* often publishes descriptions of newly described microorganisms isolated from clinical sources. Information, including biochemical reactions and sources of isolation, about new organisms of clinical importance, disease outbreaks caused by newer species, and reviews of clinical significance of certain organisms may be found in the *Annals of Internal Medicine, Journal of Infectious Diseases, Clinical Microbiology Reviews,* and *Clinical Infectious Diseases.* The data provided in these publications supplement and update *Bergey's Manual of Systematic Bacteriology,* the definitive taxonomic reference text.

Assessing Newly Described Bacteria

Since 1974, the number of genera in the family Enterobacteriaceae has increased from 12 to 28 and the number of species from 42 to more than 140, some of which have not yet been named. Similar explosions have occurred in other genera. In 1974, five species were listed in the genus *Vibrio* and four in *Campylobacter*; the genus *Legionella* was unknown. Today, there are at least 25 species in *Vibrio*, 12 *Campylobacter* species, and more than 40 species in *Legionella*. The total numbers of genera and species continue to increase dramatically.

The clinical significance of the agent of legionnaire's disease was well known long before it was isolated, characterized, and classified as *Legionella pneumophila*. In most cases, little is known about the clinical significance of a new species at the time it is first described. Assessments of clinical significance begin after clinical laboratories adopt the procedures needed to detect and identify the species and accumulate a body of data. In fact, the detection and even the identification of uncultivatable microbes from different environments are now possible using standard molecular methods. The agents of cat scratch disease (*Bartonella henselae*) and Whipple's disease (*Tropheryma whippelii*) were elucidated in this manner.

Bartonella henselae has since been cultured from several body sites from numerous patients; *T. whippelii* remains uncultivated. New species will continue to be described. Many will be able to infect humans and cause disease, especially in those individuals who are immunocompromised, burned, postsurgical, geriatric, and suffering from acquired immunodeficiency syndrome (AIDS). With today's severely immunocompromised patients, often the beneficiaries of advanced medical interventions, the concept of "pathogen" holds little meaning. Any organism is capable of causing disease in such patients under the appropriate conditions.

Role of the Clinical Laboratory

Clinical laboratory scientists should be able to isolate, identify, and determine the antimicrobial susceptibility pattern of the vast majority of human disease agents so that physicians can initiate appropriate treatment as soon as possible, and the source and means of transmission of outbreaks can be ascertained to control the disease and prevent its recurrence. The need to identify clinically relevant microorganisms both quickly and cost-effectively presents a considerable challenge. To be effective, the professional clinical laboratory staff must interact with the infectious diseases staff. Laboratory scientists should attend infectious disease rounds. They must keep abreast of new technology, equipment, and classification and should communicate this information to their medical colleagues. They should interpret, qualify, or explain laboratory reports. If a bacterial name is changed or a new species reported, the laboratory should provide background information, including a reference.

The clinical laboratory must be efficient. A concerted effort must be made to eliminate or minimize inappropriate and contaminated specimens and the performance of procedures with little or no clinical relevance. Standards for the selection, collection, and transport of specimens should be developed for both laboratory and nursing procedure manuals and reviewed periodically by a committee composed of medical, nursing, and laboratory staff. Ongoing dialogues and continuous communication with other health care workers concerning topics such as specimen collection, test selection, results interpretation, and new technology are essential to maintaining high quality microbiological services.

Biochemical and Susceptibility Testing

Most laboratories today use either commercially available miniaturized biochemical test systems or automated instruments for biochemical tests and for susceptibility testing. The kits usually contain 10 to 20 tests. The test results are converted to numerical biochemical profiles that are identified by using a codebook or a computer. Carbon source utilization systems with up to 95 tests are also available. Most identification takes 4 to 24 hours. Biochemical and enzymatic test systems for which data bases have not been developed are used by some reference laboratories.

Automated instruments can be used to identify most Gram-negative fermenters, non-fermenters, and Gram-positive bacteria, but not for anaerobes. Antimicrobial susceptibility testing can be performed for some microorganisms with this equipment, with results expressed as approximate minimum inhibitory drug concentrations. Both tasks take 4 to 24 hours. If semiautomated instruments are used, some manipulation is done manually, and the cultures (in miniature cards or microdilution plates) are incubated outside of the instrument.

The test containers are then read rapidly by the instrument, and the results are generated automatically. Instruments are also available for identification of bacteria by cell wall fatty acid profiles generated with gas-liquid chromatography (GLC), analysis of mycolic acids using high performance liquid chromatography (HPLC), and by protein-banding patterns generated by polyacrylamide gel electrophoresis (PAGE). Some other instruments designed to speed laboratory diagnosis of bacteria are those that detect (but do not identify) bacteria in blood cultures, usually faster than manual systems because of continuous monitoring. Also available are many rapid screening systems for detecting one or a series of specific bacteria, including certain streptococci, *N. meningitidis*, salmonellae, *Chlamydia trachomatis*, and many others. These screening systems are based on fluorescent antibody, agglutination, or other rapid procedures.

It is important to inform physicians as soon as a presumptive identification of an etiologic agent is obtained so that appropriate therapy can be initiated as quickly as possible. Gram stain and colony morphology; acid-fast stains; and spot indole, oxidase, and other rapid enzymatic tests may allow presumptive identification of an isolate within minutes.

Role of the Reference Laboratory

Despite recent advances, the armamentarium of the clinical laboratory is far from complete. Few laboratories can or should conduct the specialized tests that are often essential to distinguish virulent from avirulent strains. Serotyping is done only for a few species, and phage typing only rarely. Few pathogenicity tests are performed.

Not many laboratories can conduct comprehensive biochemical tests on strains that cannot be identified readily by commercially available biochemical systems. Even fewer laboratories are equipped to perform plasmid profiles, gene probes, or DNA hybridization. These and other specialized tests for the serologic or biochemical identification of some exotic bacteria, yeasts, molds, protozoans, and viruses are best done in regional reference laboratories. It is not cost-effective for smaller laboratories to store and control the quality of reagents and media for tests that are seldom run or quite complex.

In addition, it is impossible to maintain proficiency when tests are performed rarely. Sensitive methods for the epidemiologic subtyping of isolates from disease outbreaks, such as electrophoretic enzyme typing, rRNA fingerprinting, whole-cell protein electrophoretic patterns, and restriction endonuclease analysis of whole-cell or plasmid DNA, are used only in reference laboratories and a few large medical centers. Specific genetic probes are now available commercially for identifying virulence factors and many bacteria and viruses. Genetic probes are among the most common methods used for identification of *Mycobacterium tuberculosis* and *M. avium* complex in the U.S., today. Probes for *Neisseria gonorrhoeae* and *Chlamydia trachomatis* are now being used directly on clinical specimens with excellent sensitivity and almost universal specificity with same-day results. Mycobacterial probes are also being evaluated for direct specimen testing.

Interfacing with Public Health Laboratories

Hospital and local clinical laboratories interact with district, state, and federal public health laboratories in several important ways. The clinical laboratories participate in quality control and proficiency testing programmes that are conducted by federally regulated agencies. The government reference laboratories supply cultures and often reagents for use in quality control, and they conduct training programmes for clinical laboratory personnel.

All types of laboratories should interact closely to provide diagnostic services and epidemic surveillance. The primary concern of the clinical laboratory is identifying infectious disease agents and studying nosocomial and local outbreaks of disease. When the situation warrants, the local laboratory may ask the state laboratory for help in identifying an unusual organism, discovering the cause or mode of transmission in a disease outbreak, or performing specialized tests not done routinely in clinical laboratories. Cultures should be pure and should be sent on appropriate media following appropriate procedures for transport of biohazardous materials.

Pertinent information, including the type of specimen; patient name (or number), date of birth, and sex; clinical diagnosis, associated illness, date of onset, and present condition; specific agent suspected, and any other organisms isolated; relevant epidemiologic and clinical data; treatment of patient; previous laboratory results (biochemical or serologic tests); and necessary information about the submitting party must accompany each request. These data allow the state laboratory to test the specimen properly and quickly, and they provide information about occurrences within the state. For example, a food-borne outbreak might extend to many parts of the state (or beyond its boundaries). The state laboratory can alert local physicians to the possibility of such outbreaks.

Another necessary interaction between local and state laboratories is the reporting of notifiable diseases by the local laboratory. The state laboratory makes available to local laboratories summaries of the incidence of these diseases. The state laboratories also submit the summaries to the CDC weekly (or, for some diseases, yearly), and national summaries are published weekly in the*Morbidity and Mortality Weekly Report.*

Interaction between the CDC and state and federal laboratories is very similar to that between local and state laboratories. The CDC provides quality control cultures and reagents to state laboratories, and serves as a national reference laboratory for diagnostic services and epidemiologic surveillance. Local laboratories, however, must initially send specimens to the local or state public health laboratory, which, when necessary, forwards them to the CDC. The CDC reports its results back to the state laboratory, which then reports to the local laboratory.

Hazards of Clinical Laboratory Work

Clinical laboratory personnel, including support and clerical employees, are subject to the risk of infection, chemical hazards, and, in some laboratories, radioactive contamination. Such risks can be prevented or minimized by a laboratory safety programme.

Radiation Hazards

Personnel who work with radioactive materials should have taken a radioactivity safety course; they should wear radiation monitor badges and be aware of the methods for decontaminating hands, clothing, work surfaces, and equipment. They should wear gloves when working with radioactive compounds. When they work with high-level radiation, they should use a hood and stand behind a radiation shield. Preparative radioactive work should be done in a separate room with access only by personnel who are involved directly in the work.

Chemical Hazards

Chemicals can harm laboratory personnel through inhalation or skin absorption of volatile compounds; bodily contact with carcinogens, acids, bases, and other harmful chemicals; or introduction of poisonous or skin-damaging liquids into the mouth. Good laboratory practices require that volatile compounds be handled only under a hood, that hazardous chemicals never be pipetted by mouth, and that anyone working with skin-damaging chemicals wear gloves, eye guards, and other personal protective equipment as necessary. Workers should be familiar with the materials safety data sheets (MSDS) posted in an accessible place in every laboratory. These forms contain information about chemical hazards and procedures for decontamination should an accident occur.

Biologic Hazards

Microbiologic contamination is the greatest hazard in clinical microbiology laboratories. Laboratory infections are a danger not only to the clinical laboratory personnel but also to anyone else who enters the laboratory, including janitors, clerical and maintenance personnel, and visitors. The risk of infection is governed by the frequency and length of contact with the infectious agent, its virulence, the dose and route of administration, and the susceptibility of the host.

The inherent hazard of any infectious agent is affected by factors such as the volume of infectious material used, handling of the material, effectiveness of safety containment equipment, and soundness of laboratory methods. Body fluids from patients, particularly those containing blood, are considered potentially infectious for blood-borne pathogens, and must be handled appropriately.

If possible, agents that are treated differently, such as viruses as opposed to bacteria, or *M. tuberculosis* in contrast to *E. coli*, should be handled in different laboratories or in different parts of the same laboratory. When the risk category of an agent is known, it should be handled in an area with appropriate containment. All specimens sent for microbiological studies and all organisms sent to the laboratory for identification should be assumed to be potentially infectious. A separate area should be set aside for the receipt of specimens. Personnel should be aware of the potential hazards of improperly packed, broken, or leaking packages and of the proper methods for their handling and decontamination.

To prevent infection, personnel should wear moisture-proof laboratory coats at all times, wash their hands before and after wearing gloves and at the conclusion of each potential exposure to etiologic agents, refrain from mouth pipetting, and not eat, drink, smoke, or apply cosmetics in the laboratory.

Immunization may be appropriate for employees who are exposed often to certain infectious agents, including hepatitis B, yellow fever, rabies, polioviruses, meningococci, *Y. pestis*, *S. typhi*, and *Francisella tularensis*. Universal precautions, body substance isolation, and other mandated practices involve the use of personal protective equipment and engineering controls to minimize laboratory scientists' exposure to blood-borne pathogens, even when the risk of infection is unknown.

Biosafety Levels

Infectious agents are assigned to a biosafety level from 1 to 4 on the basis of their virulence.

The containment levels for organisms should correlate with the biosafety level assigned. Biosafety level 1 is for well-defined organisms not known to cause disease in healthy humans; it includes certain non-virulent *E. coli* strains (such as K-12) and *B. subtilis*.

Containment level 1 involves standard microbiologic practices, and safety equipment is not needed.

Biosafety level 2, the minimum level for clinical laboratories, is for moderate-risk agents associated with human disease.

Containment level 2 includes limited access to the work area, decontamination of all infectious wastes, use of protective gloves, and a biologic safety cabinet for use in procedures that may create aerosols.

Examples of biosafety level 2 agents include nematode, protozoan, trematode, and cestode human parasites; all human fungal pathogens except *Coccidioides immitis*; all members of the Enterobacteriaceae except *Y. pestis*; *Bacillus anthracis*; *Clostridium tetani*; *Corynebacterium diphtheriae;Haemophilus* species; leptospires; legionellae; mycobacteria other than *M. tuberculosis*; pathogenic *Neisseria* species; staphylococci, streptococci, *Treponema pallidum*; *V. cholerae*; and hepatitis and influenza viruses.

Clinical specimens potentially containing some biosafety level 3 agents, such as *Brucella* spp., are usually handled using biosafety level 2 containment practices.Biosafety level 3 is for agents that are associated with risk of serious or fatal aerosol infection.

In containment level 3, laboratory access is controlled, special clothing is worn in the laboratory, and containment equipment is used for all work with the agent. *M. tuberculosis, Coccidioides immitis, Coxiella burnetii*, and many of the arboviruses are biosafety 3 level agents.

Containment level 3 usually is recommended for work with cultures of rickettsiae, brucellae, *Y. pestis*, and a wide variety of viruses, including human immunodeficiency viruses.

Biosafety level 4 indicates dangerous and novel agents that cause diseases with high fatality rates. Maximum containment and decontamination procedures are used in containment level 4, which is found in only a few reference and research laboratories. Only a few viruses (including Lassa, Ebola, and Marburg viruses) are classified in biosafety level 4.

PROCARYOTIC LIFE

The Bacteria are a group of single-cell microorganisms with procaryotic cellular configuration. The genetic material (DNA) of procaryotic cells exists unbound in the cytoplasm of the cells.

There is no nuclear membrane, which is the definitive characteristic of eucaryotic cells such as those that make up, fungi, protista, plants and animals. Until recently, bacteria were the only known type of procaryotic cell, and the discipline of biology related to their study is called bacteriology.

In the 1980's, with the outbreak of molecular techniques applied to phylogeny of life, another group of procaryotes was defined and informally named "archaebacteria".

This group of procaryotes has since been renamed Archaea and has been awarded biological Domain status on the level with Bacteria and Eucarya. The current science of bacteriology includes the study of both domains of procaryotic cells, but the name "bacteriology" is not likely to change to reflect the inclusion of archaea in the discipline.

Actually, many archaea have been studied as intensively and as long as their bacterial counterparts, except with the notion that they were bacteria.

The derivation of Life

When life arose on Earth about 4 billion years ago, the first types of cells to evolve were procaryotic cells.

For approximately 2 billion years, procaryotic-type cells were the only form of life on Earth. The oldest known sedimentary rocks, from Greenland, are about 3.8 billion years old. The oldest known fossils are procaryotic cells, 3.5 billion years in age, found in Western Australia and South Africa. The nature of these fossils, and the chemical composition of the rocks in which they are found, indicates that lithotrophic and fermentative modes of metabolism were the first to evolve in early procaryotes. Photosynthesis developed in bacteria a bit later, at least 3 billion years ago. Anoxygenic photosynthesis (bacterial photosynthesis, which is anaerobic and does not produce O_2) preceded oxygenic photosynthesis (plant-type photosynthesis, which yields O_2).

However, oxygenic photosynthesis also arose in procaryotes, specifically in the cyanobacteria, which existed millions of years before the evolution of green algae and plants. Larger, more complicated eucaryotic cells did not appear until much later, between 1.5 and 2 billion years ago.

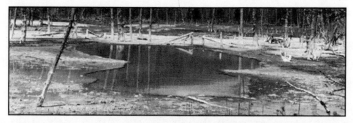

Fig. Opalescent Pool in Yellowstone National Park, Wyoming USA

The archaea and bacteria differ fundamentally in their structure from eucaryotic cells, which always contain a membrane-enclosed nucleus, multiple chromosomes, and various other membranous organelles such as mitochondria, chloroplasts, the golgi apparatus, vacuoles, etc. Unlike plants and animals, archaea and bacteria are unicellular organisms that do not develop or differentiate into multicellular forms.

Some bacteria grow in filaments or masses of cells, but each cell in the colony is identical and capable of independent existence. The cells may be adjacent to one another because they did not separate after cell division or because they remained enclosed in a common sheath or slime secreted by the cells, but typically there is no continuity or communication between the cells.

The worldwide Tree of Life

On the basis of small subunit ribosomal RNA (ssrRNA) analysis, the contemporary Tree of Life gives rise to three cellular "Domains": Archaea,Bacteria, and Eucarya. Bacteria (formerly known as eubacteria) and Archaea (formerly called archaebacteria) share the procaryotic type of cellular configuration, but otherwise are not related to one another any more closely than they are to the eucaryotic domain, Eucarya.

Between the two procaryotes, Archaea are apparently more closely related to Eucarya than are the Bacteria. Eucarya consists of all eucaryotic cell-types, including protista, fungi, plants and animals.

Most procaryotic cells are very small compared to eucaryotic cells. A typical bacterial cell is about 1 micrometer in diameter or width, while most eucaryotic cells are from 10 to 100 micrometers in diameter.

Eucaryotic cells have a much greater volume of cytoplasm and a much lower surface: volume ratio than procaryotic cells.

A typical procaryotic cell is about the size of a eucaryotic mitochondrion. Since procaryotes are too small to be seen except with the aid of a microscope, it is usually not appreciated that they are the most abundant form of life on the planet, both in terms of biomass and total numbers of species. For example, in the sea, procaryotes make up 90 per cent of the total combined weight of all organisms.

In a single gram of fertile agricultural soil there may be in excess of 10^9 bacterial cells, outnumbering all eucaryotic cells there by 10,000: 1. About 3,000 distinct species of bacteria and archaea are recognized, but this number is probably less than one per cent of all the species in nature.

These unknown procaryotes, far in excess of undiscovered or unstudied plants, are a tremendous reserve of genetic material and genetic information in nature that awaits exploitation. Procaryotes are found in all of the habitats where eucaryotes live, but, as well, in many natural environments considered too extreme or inhospitable for eucaryotic cells. Thus, the outer limits of life on Earth (hottest, coldest, driest, etc.) are usually defined by the existence of procaryotes. Where eucaryotes and procaryotes live together, there may be mutualistic associations between the organisms that allow both to survive or flourish.

The organelles of eucaryotes (mitochondria and chloroplasts) are thought to be remnants of Bacteria that invaded, or were captured by, primitive eucaryotes in the evolutionary past.

Numerous types of eucaryotic cells that exist today are inhabited by endosymbiotic procaryotes. From a metabolic standpoint, the procaryotes are extraordinarily diverse, and they exhibit several types of metabolism that are rarely or never seen in eucaryotes.

For example, the biological processes of nitrogen fixation (conversion of atmospheric nitrogen gas to ammonia) and methanogenesis (production of methane) are metabolically-unique to procaryotes and have an enormous impact on the nitrogen and carbon cycles in nature. Unique mechanisms for energy production and photosynthesis are also seen among the Archaea and Bacteria.

The lives of plants and animals are dependent upon the activities of bacterial cells. Bacteria and archaea enter into various types of symbiotic relationships with plants and animals that usually benefit both organisms, although a few bacteria are agents of disease. The metabolic activities of procaryotes in soil habitats have an enormous impact on soil fertility that can affect agricultural practices and crop yields.

In the global environment, procaryotes are absolutely essential to drive the cycles of elements that make up living systems, *i.e.*, the carbon, oxygen, nitrogen and sulfur cycles. The origins of the plant cell chloroplast and plant-type (oxygenic) photosynthesis are found in procaryotes. Most of the earth's atmospheric oxygen may have been produced by free-living bacterial cells. The bacteria fix nitrogen and a substantial amount of CO_2, as well. Bacteria or bacterial products (including their genes) can be used to increase crop yield or plant resistance to disease, or to cure or prevent plant disease.

Bacterial products include antibiotics to fight infectious disease, as well as components for vaccines used to prevent infectious disease. Because of their simplicity and our relative understanding of their biological processes, the bacteria provide convenient laboratory models for study of the molecular biology, genetics, and physiology of all types of cells, including plant and animal cells.

5

DNA of Polynucleotide Chains

The most important feature of DNA is that it is usually composed of two polynucleotide chains twisted around each other in the form of a double helix. The upper part of the figure presents the structure of the double helix shown in a schematic form. Note that if inverted 180°, the double helix looks superficially the same, due to the complementary nature of the two DNA strands.

The space-filling model of the double helix, in the lower part of the figure, shows the components of the DNA molecule and their relative positions in the helical structure. The backbone of each strand of the helix is composed of alternating sugar and phosphate residues; the bases project inward but are accessible through the major and minor grooves.

Let us begin by considering the nature of the nucleotide, the fundamental building block of DNA. The nucleotide consists of a phosphate joined to a sugar, known as 2'-deoxyribose, to which a base is attached. The sugar is called 2'-deoxyribose because there is no hydroxyl at position 2' (just two hydrogens).

Note that the positions on the ribose are designated with primes to distinguish them from positions on the bases. We can think of how the base is joined to 2'-deoxyribose by imagining the removal of a molecule of water between the hydroxyl on the 1' carbon of the sugar and the base to form a glycosidic bond.

The sugar and base alone are called a nucleoside. Likewise, we can imagine linking the phosphate to 2'-deoxyribose by removing a water molecule from between the phosphate and the hydroxyl on the 5' carbon to make a 5' phospho-monoester. Adding a phosphate (or more than one phosphate) to a nucleoside creates a nucleotide. Thus, by making a glycosidic bond between the base and the sugar, and by making a phosphoester bond between the sugar and the phosphoric acid, we have created a nucleotide. Nucleotides are, in turn, joined to each other in polynucleotide chains through the 3′ hydroxyl of 2′-deoxyribose of one nucleotide and the phosphate attached to the 5′ hydroxyl of another nucleotide.

Fig. Formation of Nucleotide by Removal of Water

This is a phosphodiester linkage in which the phosphoryl group between the two nucleotides has one sugar esterified to it through a 3′ hydroxyl and a second sugar esterified to it through a 5′ hydroxyl. Phosphodiester linkages create the repeating, sugar-phosphate backbone of the polynucleotide chain, which is a regular feature of DNA. In contrast, the order of the bases along the polynucleotide chain is irregular. This irregularity as well as the long length is, as we shall see, the basis for the enormous information content of DNA. The phosphodiester linkages impart an inherent polarity to the DNA chain. This polarity is defined by the asymmetry of the nucleotides and the way they are joined. DNA chains have a free 5′ phosphate or 5′ hydroxyl at one end and a free 3′ phosphate or 3′ hydroxyl at the other end. The convention is to write DNA sequences from the 5′ end (on the left) to the 3′ end, generally with a 5′ phosphate and a 3′ hydroxyl.

HYDROGEN BONDING

The hydrogen bonds between complementary bases are a fundamental feature of the double helix, contributing to the thermodynamic stability of the helix and providing the information content and specificity of base pairing. Hydrogen bonding might not at first glance appear to contribute importantly to the stability of DNA for the following reason. An organic molecule in aqueous solution has all of its hydrogen bonding properties satisfied by water molecules that come on and off very rapidly. As a result, for every hydrogen bond that is made when a base pair forms, a hydrogen bond with water is broken that was there before the base pair formed.

Thus, the net energetic contribution of hydrogen bonds to the stability of the double helix would appear to be modest. However, when polynucleotide strands are separate, water molecules are lined up on the bases. When strands come together in the double helix, the water molecules are displaced from the bases. This creates disorder and increases entropy, thereby stabilizing the double helix. Hydrogen bonds are not the only force that stabilizes the double helix. A second important contribution comes from stacking interactions between the bases. The bases are flat, relatively waterinsoluble molecules, and they tend to stack above each other roughly perpendicular to the direction of the helical axis.

Electron cloud interactions between bases in the helical stacks contribute significantly to the stability of the double helix. Hydrogen bonding is also important for the specificity of base pairing. Suppose we tried to pair an adenine with a cytosine. Then we would have a hydrogen bond acceptor (N_1 of adenine) lying opposite a hydrogen bond acceptor (N_3 of cytosine) with no room to put a water molecule in between to satisfy the two acceptors. Likewise, two hydrogen bond donors, the NH_2 groups at C_6 of adenine and C_4 of cytosine, would lie opposite each other. Thus, an A:C base pair would be unstable because water would have to be stripped off the donor and acceptor groups without restoring the hydrogen bond formed within the base pair.

Bases Can Flip Out from the Double Helix

As we have seen, the energetics of the double helix favour the pairing of each base on one polynucleotide strand with the complementary base on the other strand. Certain enzymes that methylate bases or remove damaged bases do so with the base in an extra helical configuration in which it is flipped out from the double helix, enabling the base to sit in the catalytic cavity of the enzyme.

Furthermore, enzymes involved in homologous recombination and DNA repair are believed to scan DNA for homology or lesions by flipping out one base after another. This is not energetically expensive because only one base is flipped out at a time. Clearly, DNA is more flexible than might be assumed at first glance.

DNA Is Usually a Right-Handed Double Helix

Applying the handedness rule from physics, we can see that each of the polynucleotide chains in the double helix is right-handed. In our mind's eye, hold our right hand up to the DNA molecule in Figure with our thumb pointing up and along the long axis of the helix and our fingers following the grooves in the helix.

Trace along one strand of the helix in the direction in which our thumb is pointing. Notice that we go around the helix in the same direction as our fingers are pointing. This does not work if we use our left hand. Try it! A consequence of the helical nature of DNA is its periodicity.

Each base pair is displaced (twisted) from the previous one by about 36°. Thus, in the X-ray crystal structure of DNA it takes a stack of about 10 base pairs to go completely around the helix (360°). That is, the helical periodicity is generally 10 base pairs per turn of the helix.

Double Helix

As a result of the double-helical structure of the two chains, the DNA molecule is a long extended polymer with two grooves that are not equal in size to each other. Why are there a minor groove and a major groove? It is a simple consequence of the geometry of the base pair. The angle at which the two sugars protrude from the base pairs (that is, the angle between the glycosidic bonds) is about 120° (for the narrow angle or 240° for the wide angle).

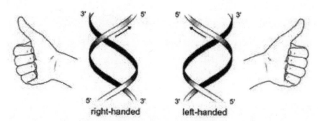

Fig. Left- and Right-Handed Helices

As a result, as more and more base pairs stack on top of each other, the narrow angle between the sugars on one edge of the base pairs generates a minor groove and the large angle on the other edge generates a major groove. (If the sugars pointed away from each other in a straight line, that is, at an angle of 180°, then two grooves would be of equal dimensions and there would be no minor and major grooves.)

Chemical Information of DNA

The edges of each base pair are exposed in the major and minor grooves, creating a pattern of hydrogen bond donors and acceptors and of van der Waals surfaces that identifies the base pair. The edge of an A:T base pair displays the following chemical groups in the following order in the major groove: a hydrogen bond acceptor (the N_7 of adenine), a hydrogen bond donor (the exocyclic amino group on C_6 of adenine), a hydrogen bond acceptor (the carbonyl group on C_4 of thymine) and a bulky hydrophobic surface (the methyl group on C_5 of thymine).

Similarly, the edge of a G:C base pair displays the following groups in the major groove: a hydrogen bond acceptor (at N_7 of guanine), a hydrogen bond acceptor (the carbonyl on C_6 of guanine), a hydrogen bond donor (the exocyclic amino group on C_4 of cytosine), a small non-polar hydrogen (the hydrogen at C_5 of cytosine).

Thus, there are characteristic patterns of hydrogen bonding and of overall shape that are exposed in the major groove that distinguish an A:T base pair from a G:C base pair, and, for that matter, A:T from T:A, and G:C from C:G. We can think of these features as a code in which A represents a hydrogen bond acceptor, D a hydrogen bond donor, M a methyl group, and H a nonpolar hydrogen. In such a code, A D A M in the major groove signifies an A:T base pair, and A A D H stands for a G:C base pair.

Likewise, M A D A stands for a T:A base pair and H D A A is characteristic of a C:G base pair. In all cases, this code of chemical groups in the major groove specifies the identity of the base pair. These patterns are important because they allow proteins to unambiguously recognize DNA sequences without having to open and thereby disrupt the double helix. Indeed, as we shall see, a principal decoding mechanism relies upon the ability of amino acid side chains to protrude into the major groove and to recognize and bind to specific DNA sequences. The minor groove is not as rich in chemical information and what information is available is less useful for distinguishing between base pairs. The small size of the minor groove is less able to accommodate amino acid side chains. Also, A:T and T:A base pairs and G:C and C:G pairs look similar to one another in the minor groove.

An A:T base pair has a hydrogen bond acceptor (at N_3 of adenine), a nonpolar hydrogen (at N_2 of adenine) and a hydrogen bond acceptor (the carbonyl on C_2 of thymine). Thus, its code is A H A. But this code is the same if read in the opposite direction, and hence an A:T base pair does not look very different from a T:A base pair from the point of view of the hydrogen bonding properties of a protein poking its side chains into the minor groove.

Likewise, a G:C base pair exhibits a hydrogen bond acceptor (at N_3 of guanine), a hydrogen bond donor (the exocyclic amino group on C_2 of guanine), and a hydrogen bond acceptor (the carbonyl on C_2 of cytosine), representing the code A D A. Thus, from the point of view of hydrogen bonding, C:G and G:C base pairs do not look very different from each other either. The minor groove does look different when comparing an A:T base pair with a G:C base pair, but G:C and C:G, or A:T and T:A, cannot be easily distinguished.

Double Helix in Multiple Conformations

Early X-ray diffraction studies of DNA, which were carried out using concentrated solutions of DNA that had been drawn out into thin fibers, revealed two kinds of structures, the B and the A forms of DNA. The B form, which is observed at high humidity, most closely corresponds to the average structure of DNA under physiological conditions. It has 10 base pairs per turn, and a wide major groove and a narrow minor groove. The A form, which is observed under conditions of low humidity, has 11 base pairs per turn. Its major groove is narrower and much deeper than that of the B form, and its minor groove is broader and shallower. The vast majority of the DNA in the cell is in the B form, but DNA does adopt the A structure in certain DNA-protein complexes. Also, as we shall see, the A form is similar to the structure that RNA adopts when double helical.

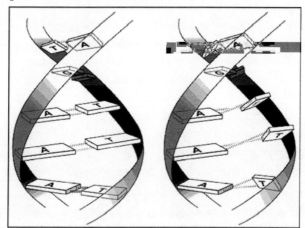

Fig. The Propeller Twist between the Purine and Pyrimidine Base Pairs of a Right-Handed Helix

The B form of DNA represents an ideal structure that deviates in two respects from the DNA in cells. First, DNA in solution, as we have seen, is somewhat more twisted on average than the B form, having on average 10.5 base pairs per turn of the helix. Second, the B form is an average structure whereas real DNA is not perfectly regular. Rather, it exhibits variations in its precise structure from base pair to base pair. This was revealed by comparison of the crystal structures of individual DNAs of different sequences. For example, the two members of each base pair do not always lie exactly in the same plane.

Rather, they can display a "propeller twist" arrangement in which the two flat bases counter rotate relative to each other along the long axis of the base pair, giving the base pair a propeller-like character. Moreover, the precise rotation per base pair is not a constant. As a result, the width of the major and minor grooves varies locally.

Thus, DNA molecules are never perfectly regular double helices. Instead, their exact conformation depends on which base pair (A:T, T:A, G:C, or C:G) is present at each position along the double helix and on the identity of neighboring base pairs. Still, the B form is for many purposes a good first approximation of the structure of DNA in cells.

DNA Can Form a Left-Handed Helix

DNA containing alternative purine and pyrimidine residues can fold into left-handed as well as right-handed helices. To understand how DNA can form a left-handed helix, we need to consider the glycosidic bond that connects the base to the 1' position of 2'-deoxyribose. This bond can be in one of two conformations called *syn* and *anti*. In right-handed DNA, the glycosidic bond is always in the *anti* conformation. In the left-handed helix, the fundamental repeating unit usually is a purine-pyrimidine dinucleotide, with the glycosidic bond in the *anti* conformation at pyrimidine residues and in the *syn* conformation at purine residues. It is this *syn* conformation at the purine nucleotides that is responsible for the left-handedness of the helix.

The change to the *syn* position in the purine residues to alternating *anti*–*syn* conformations gives the backbone of left-handed DNA a zigzag look, which distinguishes it from right-handed forms. The rotation that effects the change from *anti* to *syn* also causes the ribose group to undergo a change in its pucker. In solution alternating purine–pyrimidine residues assume the left-handed conformation only in the presence of high concentrations of positively charged ions (e.g., Na') that shield the negatively charged phosphate groups. At lower salt concentrations, they form typical right-handed conformations. The physiological significance of Z DNA is uncertain and left-handed helices probably account at most for only a small of proportion of a cell's DNA.

DNA Strands Can Separate

Because the two strands of the double helix are held together by relatively weak (non-covalent) forces, we might expect that the two strands could come apart easily. Indeed, the original structure for the double helix suggested that DNA replication would occur in just this manner. The complementary strands of double helix can also be made to come apart when a solution of DNA is heated above physiological temperatures (to near 100°C) or under conditions of high pH, a process known as denaturation.

However, this complete separation of DNA strands by denaturation is reversible. When heated solutions of denatured DNA are slowly cooled, single strands often meet their complementary strands and reform regular double helices. The capacity to renature denatured DNA molecules permits artificial hybrid DNA molecules to be formed by slowly cooling mixtures of denatured DNA from two different sources. Likewise, hybrids can be formed between complementary strands of DNA and RNA.

The ability to form hybrids between two single-stranded nucleic acids (hybridization) is the basis for several indispensable techniques in molecular biology, such as Southern blot hybridization and DNA microarrays. Important insights into the properties of the double helix were obtained from classic experiments carried out in the 1950s in which the denaturation of DNA was studied under a variety of conditions.

In these experiments DNA denaturation was monitored by measuring the absorbance of ultraviolet light passed through a solution of DNA. DNA maximally absorbs ultraviolet light at a wavelength of about 260 nm. It is the bases that are principally responsible for this absorption. When the temperature of a solution of DNA is raised to near the boiling point of water, the optical density (absorbance) at 260 nm markedly increases.

The explanation for this increase is that duplex DNA is hypochromic; it absorbs less ultraviolet light by about 40% than do individual DNA chains. The hypochromicity is due to base stacking, which diminishes the capacity of the bases in duplex DNA to absorb ultraviolet light.

If we plot the optical density of DNA as a function of temperature, we observe that the increase in absorption occurs abruptly over a relatively narrow temperature range. The midpoint of this transition is the melting point or Tm. Like ice, DNA melts: it undergoes a transition from a highly ordered double-helical structure to a much less ordered structure of individual strands.

The sharpness of the increase in absorbance at the melting temperature tells us that the denaturation and renaturation of complementary DNA strands is a highly cooperative, zippering-like process.

Renaturation, for example, probably occurs by means of a slow nucleation process in which a relatively small stretch of bases on one strand find and pair with their complement on the complementary strand. The remainder of the two strands then rapidly zipper-up from the nucleation site to reform an extended double helix.

The melting temperature of DNA is a characteristic of each DNA that is largely determined by the G:C content of the DNA and the ionic strength of the solution. The higher the percent of G:C base pairs in the DNA (and hence the lower the content of A:T base pairs), the higher the melting point. Likewise, the higher the salt concentration of the solution the greater the temperature at which the DNA denatures.

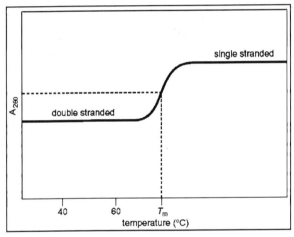

Fig. DNA Denaturation Curve

How do we explain this behaviour? G:C base pairs contribute more to the stability of DNA than do A:T base pairs because of the greater number of hydrogen bonds for the former (three in a G:C base pair versus two for A:T) but also importantly because the stacking interactions of G:C base pairs with adjacent base pairs are more favorable than the corresponding interactions of A:T base pairs with their neighboring base pairs.

The effect of ionic strength reflects another fundamental feature of the double helix. The backbones of the two DNA strands contain phosphoryl groups, which carry a negative charge. These negative charges are close enough across the two strands that if not shielded they tend to cause the strands to repel each other, facilitating their separation. At high ionic strength, the negative charges are shielded by cations, thereby stabilizing the helix. Conversely, at low ionic strength the unshielded negative charges render the helix less stable.

CIRCLES CIRCULAR DNA MOLECULES

It was initially believed that all DNA molecules are linear and have two free ends. Indeed, the chromosomes of eukaryotic cells each contain a single (extremely long) DNA molecule. But now we know that some DNAs are circles. For example, the chromosome of the small monkey DNA virus SV40 is a circular, double-helical DNA molecule of about 5,000 base pairs. Also, most (but not all) bacterial chromosomes are circular; *E. coli* has a circular chromosome of about 5 million base pairs.

Additionally, many bacteria have small autonomously replicating genetic elements known as plasmids, which are generally circular DNA molecules. Interestingly, some DNA molecules are sometimes linear and sometimes circular. The most well-known example is that of the bacteriophage ', a DNA virus of *E. coli*. The phage ' genome is a linear double-stranded molecule in the virion particle. However, when the ' genome is injected into an *E. coli* cell during infection, the DNA circularizes. This occurs by base-pairing between single-stranded regions that protrude from the ends of the DNA and that have complementary sequences ("sticky ends").

DNA Topology

As DNA is a flexible structure, its exact molecular parameters are a function of both the surrounding ionic environment and the nature of the DNA-binding proteins with which it is complexed. Because their ends are free, linear DNA molecules can freely rotate to accommodate changes in the number of times the two chains of the double helix twist about each other. But if the two ends are covalently linked to form a circular DNA molecule and if there are no interruptions in the sugar phosphate backbones of the two strands, then the absolute number of times the chains can twist about each other cannot change. Such a covalently closed, circular DNA is said to be topologically constrained.

Even the linear DNA molecules of eukaryotic chromosomes are subject to topological constraints due to their entrainment in chromatin and interaction with other cellular components. Despite these constraints, DNA participates in numerous dynamic processes in the cell. For example, the two strands of the double helix, which are twisted around each other, must rapidly separate in order for DNA to be duplicated and to be transcribed into RNA. Thus, understanding the topology of DNA and how the cell both accommodates and exploits topological constraints during DNA replication, transcription, and other chromosomal transactions is of fundamental importance in molecular biology.

Circular DNA

Let us consider the topological properties of covalently closed, circular DNA, which is referred to as cccDNA. Because there are no interruptions in either polynucleotide chain, the two strands of cccDNA cannot be separated from each other without the breaking of a covalent bond. If we wished to separate the two circular strands without permanently breaking any bonds in the sugar phosphate backbones,we would have to pass one strand through the other strand repeatedly(we will encounter an enzyme that can perform just this feat!).

The number of times one strand would have to be passed through the other strand in order for the two strands to be entirely separated from each other is called the linking number. The linking number, which is always an integer, is an invariant topological property of cccDNA, no matter how much the DNA molecule is distorted.

Linking Number Is Composed of Twist and Writhe

The linking number is the sum of two geometric components called the twist and the writhe. Let us consider twist first. Twist is simply the number of helical turns of one strand about the other, that is, the number of times one strand completely wraps around the other strand. Consider a cccDNA that is lying flat on a plane. In this flat conformation, the linking number is fully composed of twist. Indeed, the twist can be easily determined by counting the number of times the two strands cross each other. The helical crossovers (twist) in a right-handed helix are defined as positive such that the linking number of DNA will have a positive value. But cccDNA is generally not lying flat on a plane.

Rather, it is usually torsionally stressed such that the long axis of the double helix crosses over itself, often repeatedly, in three-dimensional space. This is called *writhe*. To visualize the distortions caused by torsional stress, think of the coiling of a telephone cord that has been overtwisted. Writhe can take two forms.

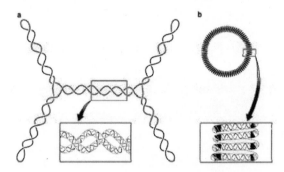

Fig. Two Forms of Writhe of Supercoiled DNA

One form is the interwound or plectonemic writhe, in which the long axis is twisted around itself. The other form of writhe is a toroid or spiral in which the long axis is wound in a cylindrical manner, as often occurs when DNA wraps around protein. The writhing number (*Wr*) is the total number of interwound and/or spiral writhes in cccDNA. For example, the molecule has a writhe of 4 from 4 interwound writhes. Interwound writhe and spiral writhe are topologically equivalent to each other and are readily interconvertible geometric properties of cccDNA.

Also, twist and writhe are interconvertible. A molecule of cccDNA can readily undergo distortions that convert some of its twist to writhe or some of its writhe to twist without the breakage of any covalent bonds.

The only constraint is that the sum of the twist number (*Tw*) and the writhing number (*Wr*) must remain equal to the linking number (*Lk*). This constraint is described by the equation: *Lk = Tw + Wr*.

Negative Supercoiling in Eukaryotes

DNA in the nucleus of eukaryotic cells is packaged in small particles known as nucleosomes in which the double helix is wrapped almost two times around the outside circumference of a protein core. We will be able to recognize this wrapping as the toroid or spiral form of writhe. Importantly, it occurs in a lefthanded manner.. It turns out that writhe in the form of left-handed spirals is equivalent to negative supercoils. Thus, the packaging of DNA into nucleosomes introduces negative superhelical density.

Topoisomerases Can Relax Supercoiled DNA

As we have seen, the linking number is an invariant property of DNA that is topologically constrained. It can only be changed by introducing interruptions into the sugar-phosphate backbone. A remarkable class of enzymes known as topoisomerases are able to do just that by introducing transient nicks or breaks into the DNA. Topoisomerases are of two broad types. Type II topoisomerases change the linking number in steps of two. They make transient double-stranded breaks in the DNA, through which they pass a region of uncut duplex DNA before resealing the break. Type II topoisomerases require energy from ATP hydrolysis for their action. Type I topoisomerases, in contrast, change the linking number of DNA in steps of one. They make transient singlestranded breaks in the DNA, allowing one strand to pass through the break in the other before resealing the nick. Type I topoisomerases relax DNA by removing supercoils (dissipating writhe).

They can be compared to the protocol of introducing nicks into cccDNA with DNase and then repairing the nicks, which as we saw can be used to relax cccDNA, except that type I topoisomerases relax DNA in a controlled and concerted manner. In contrast to type II topoisomerases, type I topoisomerases do not require ATP. Both type I and type II topoisomerases work through an intermediate in which the enzyme is covalently attached to one end of the broken DNA.

Special Topoisomerase

Both prokaryotes and eukaryotes have type I and type II topoisomerases, which are capable of removing supercoils from DNA. In addition, however, prokaryotes have a special type II topoisomerase known as DNA gyrase that is able to introduce negative supercoils, rather than remove them.

DNA gyrase is responsible for the negative supercoiling of chromosomes in prokaryotes, which facilitates unwinding of the DNA duplex during transcription and DNA replication.

DNA TOPOISOMERS

Covalently closed, circular DNA molecules of the same length but of different linking numbers are called DNA topoisomers. Even though topoisomers have the same molecular weight, they can be separated from each other by electrophoresis through a gel of agarose. The basis for this separation is that the greater the writhe the more compact the shape of a cccDNA. Once again, think of how supercoiling a telephone cord causes it to become more compact. The more compact the DNA, the more easily (up to a point) it is able to migrate through the gel matrix.

Thus, a fully relaxed cccDNA migrates more slowly than a highly supercoiled topoisomer of the same circular DNA. Figure shows a ladder of

DNA topoisomers resolved by gel electrophoresis. Molecules in adjacent rungs of the ladder differ from each other by a linking number difference of just one. Obviously, electrophoretic mobility is highly sensitive to the topological state of DNA.

DNA Has a Helical Periodicity

The observation that DNA topoisomers can be separated from each other electrophoretically is the basis for a simple experiment that proves that DNA has a helical periodicity of about 10.5 base pairs per turn in solution. Consider three cccDNAs of sizes 3990, 3995, and 4011 base pairs that were relaxed to completion by treatment with topoisomerase I. When subjected to electrophoresis through agarose, the 3990- and 4011-base-pair DNAs exhibit essentially identical mobilities.

Due to thermal fluctuation, topoisomerase treatment actually generates a narrow spectrum of topoisomers, but for simplicity let us consider the mobility of only the most abundant topoisomer (that corresponding to the cccDNA in its most relaxed state). The mobilities of the most abundant topoisomers for the 3990- and 4011-base-pair DNAs are indistinguishable because the 21-base-pair difference between them is negligible compared to the sizes of the rings.

The most abundant topoisomer for the 3995-base-pair ring, however, is found to migrate slightly more rapidly than the other two rings even though it is only 5 base pairs larger than the 3990-base-pair ring. How are we to explain this anomaly? The 3990- and 4011- base-pair rings in their most relaxed states are expected to have linking numbers equal to Lk^O, that is, 380 in the case of the 3990-base-pair ring (dividing the size by 10.5 base pairs) and 382 in the case of the 4011-base-pair ring. Because Lk is equal to Lk^O, the linking difference ($'Lk = Lk - Lk^O$) in both cases is zero and there is no writhe.

But because the linking number must be an integer, the most relaxed state for the 3995-base-pair ring would be either of two topoisomers having linking numbers of 380 or 381. However, Lk^O for the 3995-base-pair ring is 380.5. Thus, even in its most relaxed state, a covalently closed circle of 3995 base pairs would necessarily have about half a unit of writhe (its linking difference would be 0.5), and hence it would migrate more rapidly than the 3990- and 4011-base-pair circles.

In other words, to explain how rings that differ in length by 21 base pairs (two turns of the helix) have the same mobility whereas a ring that differs in length by only 5 base pairs (about half a helical turn) exhibits a different mobility, we must conclude that DNA in solution has a helical periodicity of about 10.5 base pairs per turn.

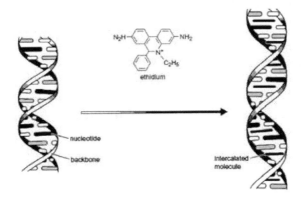

Fig. Intercalation of Ethidium Bromide into DNA

Ethidium Ions Cause DNA to Unwind

Ethidium is a large, flat, multi-ringed cation. Its planar shape enables ethidium to slip (intercalate) between the stacked base pairs of DNA. Because it fluoresces when exposed to ultraviolet light, and because its fluorescence increases dramatically after intercalation, ethidium is used as a stain to visualize DNA. When an ethidium ion intercalates between two base pairs, it causes the DNA to unwind by 26°, reducing the normal rotation per base pair from ~36° to ~10°. In other words, ethidium decreases the twist of DNA.

Imagine the extreme case of a DNA molecule that has an ethidium ion between every base pair. Instead of 10 base pairs per turn it would have 36! When ethidium binds to linear DNA or to a nicked circle, it simply causes the helical pitch to increase. But consider what happens when ethidium binds to covalently closed, circular DNA.

The linking number of the cccDNA does not change (no covalent bonds are broken and resealed), but the twist decreases by 26° for each molecule of ethidium that has bound to the DNA. Because $Lk = Tw + Wr$, this decrease in Tw must be compensated for by a corresponding increase in Wr. If the circular DNA is initially negatively supercoiled (as is normally the case for circular DNAs isolated from cells), then the addition of ethidium will increase Wr. In other words, the addition of ethidium will relax the DNA.

If enough ethidium is added, the negative supercoiling will be brought to zero, and if even more ethidium is added, Wr will increase above zero and the DNA will become positively supercoiled. Because the binding of ethidium increases *Wr*, its presence greatly affects the migration of cccDNA during gel electrophoresis. In the presence of non-saturating amounts of ethidium, negatively supercoiled circular DNAs are more relaxed and migrate more slowly, whereas relaxed cccDNAs become positively supercoiled and migrate more rapidly.

DNA AND MOLECULAR GENETICS

The physical carrier of inheritance

While the period from the early 1900s to World War II has been considered the "golden age" of genetics, scientists still had not determined that DNA, and not protein, was the hereditary material. However, during this time a great many genetic discoveries were made and the link between genetics and evolution was made.

Friedrich Meischer in 1869 isolated DNA from fish sperm and the pus of open wounds. Since it came from nuclei, Meischer named this new chemical, nuclein. Subsequently the name was changed to nucleic acid and lastly to deoxyribonucleic acid (DNA). Robert Feulgen, in 1914, discovered that fuchsin dye stained DNA. DNA was then found in the nucleus of all eukaryotic cells.

During the 1920s, biochemist P.A. Levene analyzed the components of the DNA molecule. He found it contained four nitrogenous bases: cytosine, thymine, adenine, and guanine; deoxyribose sugar; and a phosphate group. He concluded that the basic unit (nucleotide) was composed of a base attached to a sugar and that the phosphate also attached to the sugar.

He (unfortunately) also erroneously concluded that the proportions of bases were equal and that there was a tetranucleotide that was the repeating structure of the molecule. The nucleotide, however, remains as the fundemantal unit (monomer) of the nucleic acid polymer. There are four nucleotides: those with cytosine (C), those with guanine (G), those with adenine (A), and those with thymine (T).

During the early 1900s, the study of genetics began in earnest: the link between Mendel's work and that of cell biologists resulted in the chromosomal theory of inheritance; Garrod proposed the link between genes and "inborn errors of metabolism"; and the question was formed: what is a gene? The answer came from the study of a deadly infectious disease: pneumonia. During the 1920s Frederick Griffith studied the difference between a disease-causing strain of the pneumonia causing bacteria (*Streptococcus peumoniae*) and a strain that did not cause pneumonia.

The pneumonia-causing strain (the S strain) was surrounded by a capsule. The other strain (the R strain) did not have a capsule and also did not cause pneumonia. Frederick Griffith was able to induce a nonpathogenic strain of the bacterium *Streptococcus pneumoniae* to become pathogenic. Griffith referred to a transforming factor that caused the non-pathogenic bacteria to become pathogenic.

Griffith injected the different strains of bacteria into mice. The S strain killed the mice; the R strain did not. He further noted that if heat killed S strain was injected into a mouse, it did not cause pneumonia. When he combined heat-killed S with Live R and injected the mixture into a mouse (remember neither alone will kill the mouse) that the mouse developed pneumonia and died. Bacteria recovered from the mouse had a capsule and killed other mice when injected into them!

Hypotheses:

- The dead S strain had been reanimated/resurrected.
- The Live R had been transformed into Live S by some "transforming factor".

Further experiments led Griffith to conclude that number 2 was correct.

In 1944, Oswald Avery, Colin MacLeod, and Maclyn McCarty revisited Griffith's experiment and concluded the transforming factor was DNA. Their evidence was strong but not totally conclusive. The then-current favourite for the hereditary material was protein; DNA was not considered by many scientists to be a strong candidate.

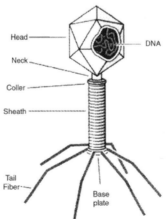

Fig. **Structure of a Bacteriophage Virus**

The breakthrough in the quest to determine the hereditary material came from the work of Max Delbruck and Salvador Luria in the 1940s.

Bacteriophage are a type of virus that attacks bacteria, the viruses that Delbruck and Luria worked with were those attacking *Escherichia coli,* a bacterium found in human intestines. Bacteriophages consist of protein coats covering DNA. Bacteriophages infect a cell by injecting DNA into the host cell. This viral DNA then "disappears" while taking over the bacterial machinery and beginning to make new virus instead of new bacteria. After 25 minutes the host cell bursts, releasing hundreds of new bacteriophage.

Phages have DNA and protein, making them ideal to resolve the nature of the hereditary material. In 1952, Alfred D. Hershey and Martha Chase conducted a series of experiments to determine whether protein or DNA was the hereditary material. By labeling the DNA and protein with different (and mutually exclusive) radioisotopes, they would be able to determine which chemical (DNA or protein) was getting into the bacteria.

Such material must be the hereditary material (Griffith's transforming agent). Since DNA contains Phosphorous (P) but no Sulfur (S), they tagged the DNA with radioactive Phosphorous-32. Conversely, protein lacks P but does have S, thus it could be tagged with radioactive Sulfur-35. Hershey and Chase found that the radioactive S remained outside the cell while the radioactive P was found inside the cell, indicating that DNA was the physical carrier of heredity.

The Structure of DNA

Erwin Chargaff analyzed the nitrogenous bases in many different forms of life, concluding that the amount of purines does not always equal the amount of pyrimidines (as proposed by Levene). DNA had been proven as the genetic material by the Hershey-Chase experiments, but how DNA served as genes was not yet certain. DNA must carry information from parent cell to daughter cell. It must contain information for replicating itself. It must be chemically stable, relatively unchanging.

However, it must be capable of mutational change. Without mutations there would be no process of evolution. Many scientists were interested in deciphering the structure of DNA, among them were Francis Crick, James Watson, Rosalind Franklin, and Maurice Wilkens. Watson and Crick gathered all available data in an attempt to develop a model of DNA structure. Franklin took X-ray diffraction photomicrographs of crystalline DNA extract, the key to the puzzle. The data known at the time was that DNA was a long molecule, proteins were helically coiled (as determined by the work of Linus Pauling), Chargaff's base data, and the x-ray diffraction data of Franklin and Wilkens.

DNA is a double helix, with bases to the centre (like rungs on a ladder) and sugar-phosphate units along the sides of the helix (like the sides of a twisted ladder). The strands are complementary (deduced by Watson and Crick from Chargaff's data, A pairs with T and C pairs with G, the pairs held together by hydrogen bonds). Notice that a double-ringed purine is always bonded to a single ring pyrimidine.

Purines are Adenine (A) and Guanine (G). We have encountered Adenosine triphosphate (ATP) before, although in that case the sugar was ribose, whereas in DNA it is deoxyribose. Pyrimidines are Cytosine (C) and Thymine (T). The bases are complementary, with A on one side of the molecule we only get T on the other side, similarly with G and C. If we know the base sequence of one strand we know its complement.

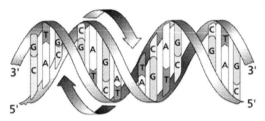

Fig. The Ribbon Model of DNA

DNA Replication

DNA was proven as the hereditary material and Watson et al. had deciphered its structure. What remained was to determine how DNA copied its information and how that was expressed in the phenotype. Matthew Meselson and Franklin W. Stahl designed an experiment to determine the method of DNA replication. Three models of replication were considered likely.

- *Conservative replication:* Would somehow produce an entirely new DNA strand during replication.

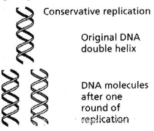

Fig. Conservative Model of DNA Replication

- *Semiconservative Replication:* Would produce two DNA molecules, each of which was composed of one-half of the parental DNA along with an entirely new complementary strand. In other words the new DNA would consist of one new and one old strand of DNA. The existing strands would serve as complementary templates for the new strand.

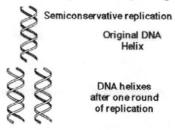

Semiconservative replication

Original DNA
Helix

DNA helixes
after one round
of replication

Fig. **The Semiconservative Model of DNA Structure**

- *Dispersive replication:* Involved the breaking of the parental strands during replication, and somehow, a reassembly of molecules that were a mix of old and new fragments on each strand of DNA.

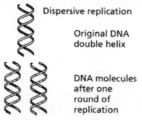

Dispersive replication

Original DNA
double helix

DNA molecules
after one
round of
replication

Fig. **The Dispersive Replication Model of DNA Replication**

The Mesclson-Stahl experiment involved the growth of *E. coli* bacteria on a growth medium containing heavy nitrogen (Nitrogen-15 as opposed to the more common, but lighter molecular weight isotope, Nitrogen-14). The first generation of bacteria was grown on a medium where the sole source of N was Nitrogen-15.

The bacteria were then transferred to a medium with light (Nitrogen-14) medium. Watson and Crick had predicted that DNA replication was semi-conservative. If it was, then the DNA produced by bacteria grown on light medium would be intermediate between heavy and light. It was. DNA replication involves a great many building blocks, enzymes and a great deal of ATP energy (remember that after the S phase of the cell cycle cells have a G phase to regenerate energy for cell division).

Only occurring in a cell once per (cell) generation, DNA replication in humans occurs at a rate of 50 nucleotides per second, 500/second in prokaryotes. Nucleotides have to be assembled and available in the nucleus, along with energy to make bonds between nucleotides.

DNA polymerases unzip the helix by breaking the H-bonds between bases. Once the polymerases have opened the molecule, an area known as the replication bubble forms (always initiated at a certain set of nucleotides, the origin of replication). New nucleotides are placed in the fork and link to the corresponding parental nucleotide already there (A with T, C with G). Prokaryotes open a single replication bubble, while eukaryotes have multiple bubbles. The entire length of the DNA molecule is replicated as the bubbles meet.

Since the DNA strands are antiparallel, and replication proceeds in thje 5' to 3' direction on EACH strand, one strand will form a continuous copy, while the other will form a series of short Okazaki fragments.

ENZYME STRUCTURE PROVIDES CLUES TO DNA

Before a cell can begin to divide or differentiate, the genetic information within the cell's DNA must be copied, or "transcribed," onto complementary strands of RNA. RNA polymerase II (pol II) is an enzyme that, by itself, can unwind the DNA double helix, synthesize RNA, and proofread the result. When combined with other molecules that regulate and control the transcription process, pol II is the key to successful interpretion of an organism's genetic code.

However, the size, complexity, scarcity, and fragility of pol II complexes have made analysis of these macromolecules by x-ray crystallography a formidable challenge. A team of structural biologists has met this challenge using data obtained from both the Stanford Synchrotron Radiation Laboratory and the Macromolecular Crystallography Facility at the ALS. The resultant high-resolution model of a 10-subunit pol II complex suggests roles for each of the subunits and will allow researchers to begin unraveling the intricacies of DNA transcription and its role in gene expression.

In this work, the researchers studied the pol II enzyme from the yeast *Saccharomyces cerevisiae*, which is likely to be an excellent model for the human enzyme in light of its highly similar gene sequences. It is also the best-characterized form of the pol II enzyme, having been the subject of many biochemical and low-resolution structural studies in the past.

To obtain a high-resolution structure, the research team drew on its considerable expertise in the preparation of protein crystals: two-dimensional crystals of pol II (minus two small subunits found to impede crystal growth) were used as seeds for growing three-dimensional crystals. These crystals, when produced in an inert atmosphere to prevent oxidation, enabled the collection of data to 3.5-angstrom resolution. The addition of a final soaking procedure to produce uniform crystals, combined with high-brightness x-ray sources, resulted in a resolution of 3.0 angstroms.

The current results bring into focus the somewhat fuzzy features previously observed in or inferred from earlier experiments. More importantly, the structural details suggest possible explanations for some of the unusual characteristics of this enzyme, which include a high processivity (the ability to synthesize very long strands of RNA) and the tendency to work in periodic spurts separated by pauses.

While it is known that additional proteins (transcription factors) play a role in controlling the activity of pol II (for example, restarting after a pause), scientists have yet to understand how such proteins interact with pol II binding sites to perform their various functions. The pol II model reported here establishes the positions of the various subunits and provides detailed information about the DNA/RNA binding domains.

The data reveal two main subunits (Rpb1 and Rpb2) separated by a deep cleft where DNA can enter the complex. At the end of the cleft is the active site, where the DNA can be unwound for a short distance (the "transcription bubble") and a DNA/RNA hybrid can be produced. Two prominent grooves lead away from the active site, either of which could accommodate the exiting RNA transcript. An opening below the active site may allow the entry of nucleotides (for manufacturing RNA) and transcription factors (for regulating the process). The same opening may provide room for the leading end of the RNA strand during "backtracking" maneuvers, which are important for proofreading and for traversing obstacles such as DNA damage.

Other notable features that might help account for the great stability of this transcribing complex include a pair of "jaws" that appear to grip the DNA strands as they enter the complex and, closer to the active site, a clamp on the DNA that could possibly be locked in the closed position by the presence of RNA.

The high-resolution pol II structure reported here is a landmark achievement, pulling together threads from numerous diverse research efforts into a cohesive whole. Further study should yield many new insights into the detailed mechanisms of pol II and its transcription factors. Construction of an atomic model is already well underway.

UNRAVELING DNA

Encoded into the double-helical strands of DNA, the human genome is the complete set of instructions required to make a human being. While the mapping of the human genome (roughly three billion components) is certainly a Herculean accomplishment, it is only the first step toward realizing the full potential of genomic medicine in the diagnosis, monitoring, and treatment of disease. Beyond knowing what the genetic blueprint says, scientists must understand how that blueprint gets interpreted, or "expressed" as an individual with unique traits. The pol II enzyme is the catalyst for a major step in this process.

As a pol II molecule slides along a DNA molecule, it "unzips" the strands of the DNA double helix, synthesizes a complementary strand of RNA (which will carry the genetic information to where it is needed), and verifies that no mistakes have occurred. This process is regulated by transcription factors— separate molecules that bind to pol II and determine which genes are expressed, at what stage of development, and in which tissue.

Done correctly, this process results in healthy cell growth and differentiation; otherwise, aberrations such as cancer can be the result. Thus, details of the structure of pol II, including information about its binding sites and how they interact with transcription factors, will provide valuable insight into the detailed mechanisms underlying the flow of genetic information from DNA to RNA to protein, which is necessary for life and health.

EACH BASE HAS ITS PREFERRED TAUTOMERIC FORM

The bases in DNA fall into two classes, purines and pyrimidines. The purines are adenine and guanine, and the pyrimidines are cytosine and thymine. The purines are derived from the double-ringed structure. Adenine and guanine share this essential structure but with different groups attached. Likewise, cytosine and thymine are variations on the single-ringed structure shown in Figure. The numbering of the positions in the purine and pyrimidine rings. The bases are attached to the deoxyribose by glycosidic linkages at N_1 of the pyrimidines or at N9 of the purines.

Each of the bases exists in two alternative tautomeric states, which are in equilibrium with each other. The equilibrium lies far to the side of the conventional structures shown in Figure, which are the predominant states and the ones important for base pairing.

The nitrogen atoms attached to the purine and pyrimidine rings are in the amino form in the predominant state and only rarely assume the imino configuration. Likewise, the oxygen atoms attached to the guanine and thymine normally have the keto form and only rarely take on the enol configuration. As examples, tautomerization of cytosine into the imino form

(a) and guanine into the enol form (b). As we shall see, the capacity to form an alternative tautomer is a frequent source of errors during DNA synthesis.

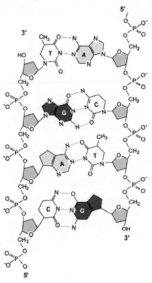

Fig. Detailed Structure of Polynucleotide Polymer

STRANDS OF THE DOUBLE HELIX

The double helix is composed of two polynucleotide chains that are held together by weak, non-covalent bonds between pairs of bases. Adenine on one chain is always paired with thymine on the other chain and, likewise, guanine is always paired with cytosine. The two strands have the same helical geometry but base pairing holds them together with the opposite polarity.

That is, the base at the 5' end of one strand is paired with the base at the 3' end of the other strand. The strands are said to have an anti-parallel orientation. This anti-parallel orientation is a stereochemical consequence of the way that adenine and thymine and guanine and cytosine pair with each together.

Chains of the Double Helix

The pairing between adenine and thymine and between guanine and cytosine results in a complementary relationship between the sequence of bases on the two intertwined chains and gives DNA its self-encoding character. For example, if we have the sequence 5'-ATGTC-3' on one chain, the opposite chain must have the complementary sequence 3'-TACAG-5'. The strictness of the rules for this "Watson-Crick" pairing derives from the complementarity both of shape and of hydrogen bonding properties between adenine and thymine and between guanine and cytosine.

Adenine and thymine match up so that a hydrogen bond can form between the exocyclic amino group at C_6 on adenine and the carbonyl at C_4 in thymine; and likewise, a hydrogen bond can form between N1 of adenine and N_3 of thymine.

Fig. The Figure shows Hydrogen Bonding between the Bases

A corresponding arrangement can be drawn between a guanine and a cytosine, so that there is both hydrogen bonding and shape complementarity in this base pair as well. A G:C base pair has three hydrogen bonds, because the exocyclic NH_2 at C_2 on guanine lies opposite to, and can hydrogen bond with, a carbonyl at C_2 on cytosine. Likewise, a hydrogen bond can form between N_1 of guanine and N_3 of cytosine and between the carbonyl at C_6 of guanine and the exocyclic NH_2 at C_4 of cytosine.

Watson-Crick base pairing requires that the bases are in their preferred tautomeric states. An important feature of the double helix is that the two base pairs have exactly the same geometry; having an A:T base pair or a G:C base pair between the two sugars does not perturb the arrangement of the sugars. Neither does T:A or C:G. In other words, there is an approximately twofold axis of symmetry that relates the two sugars and all four base pairs can be accommodated within the same arrangement without any distortion of the overall structure of the DNA.

6

The Genetic Code of DNA Structure

The structure of DNA encodes all the information every cell needs to function and thrive. In addition, DNA carries hereditary information in a form that can be copied and passed intact from generation to generation. A gene is a segment of DNA. The biochemical instructions found within most genes, known as the genetic code, specify the chemical structure of a particular protein. Proteins are composed of long chains of amino acids, and the specific sequence of these amino acids dictates the function of each protein. The DNA structure of a gene determines the arrangement of amino acids in a protein, ultimately determining the type and function of the protein manufactured.

GENETICS DISORDERS

Schizophrenia is one of the more complex and less understood of the psychological disorders. For many years, studies have explored the genetic aspect of this syndrome in an effort to provide a better understanding of its etiology, symptoms, course, and development. Much of what is involved in schizophrenia still remains unclear, although great strides have been accomplished by research in the area.

In trying to understand the etiology of psychiatric disorders, one cannot avoid studying gene—environment interactions. Just as genes influence the susceptibility of an individual to the development of almost any disorder, environmental factors are also seen as important etiological contributors to disturbance. Consequently, whether or not genetic or environmental variation is involved in the development of schizophrenia is no longer considered to be an important point of contention in this area of research.

Instead, most of the current investigations appear to be concerned with acquiring a more thorough understanding of the magnitude and relevance of both environmental and genetic variation and the ways in which these interact to establish the various manifestations of schizophrenia.

Today there seems to be little doubt that a genetic basis for schizophrenia exists. However, the specific schizophrenia-producing genetic components and the method by which they are transmitted remain unclear. Genetic investigations have involved primarily three methodologies: family studies, twin studies, and adoption studies. Despite some difficulties, these methods have obtained strong evidence pointing toward the involvement of genetic factors in the development of schizophrenia. Currently, the amount of interest and speculation in this area of research is high, and on the basis of findings, sophisticated models and new, more innovative research techniques are being developed.

The major conceptual, diagnostic, and methodological difficulties inherent in this area of investigation, the evidence for the existence of genetic factors in the etiology of schizophrenia, and the models for a genetic mode of transmission that have arisen from these lines of research.

One of the more difficult aspects of this field remains the lack of knowledge concerning the nature of schizophrenia. To date, no homogeneous group of schizophrenics has been isolated and no unitary etiology for the disorder has been found.

The possibility exists that schizophrenia is not a single, unitary disorder, but may consist of a number of different entities. Schizophrenic heterogeneity could be present at several levels. Seemingly similar phenotypic expressions may be due to quite different etiologies. As a result, the reliance upon symptomatology for the differentiation of schizophrenic subtypes may be grossly misleading. To complicate matters further, the complexity of gene operations makes it difficult to delineate the various interacting etiological components of a schizophrenic disorder.

The nature of the activating environment and the timing of that activation in addition to the gene could all combine to produce a single phenotype. Therefore, a range of possible phenotypic outcomes exists for every gene as a function of the activating environment and the time of activation. Depending on the environmental circumstances, there are a number of different genes that can produce a single phenotype. Consequently, several genetic mechanisms may underlie the expression of a single characteristic.

If schizophrenia is in fact heterogeneous, many of the present research strategies may prove inadequate because most rely on the implicit assumption of homogeneity among patients studied. A schizophrenic sample based on an overinclusive diagnostic category would result in variable schizophrenic performance. As a result, common findings among schizophrenics would be difficult to detect and valid hypotheses may be prematurely discarded on the basis that the data fail to meet statistical significance.

The failure to reach a clear consensus on the nature of schizophrenia has resulted in conflicting viewpoints. To date, genetic studies of schizophrenia have relied almost exclusively on the assumption of a model in which schizophrenia consists of a complex disorder amenable to the same type of study and displaying the same pathogenic characteristics as an inheritable disease.

Other points of view, especially those among the psychodynamic and contextualist schools of thought, hold that the conceptualization of schizophrenia as a disease entity is inadequate and unjustified. For example, Sarbin and Mancuso claim that schizophrenia is a label and the product of social processes resulting in the imposition of a moral verdict in response to certain undesirable Behaviours. Others have proposed that certain forms of familial interaction predispose an individual to schizophrenia, whereas still others have preferred to focus on the schizophrenic's intrapsychic world and dynamics. An interesting model postulated by Meehl incorporates both genetic and environmental factors to explain the occurrence of schizophrenia. Meehl suggests that all that is inherited in schizophrenia is an integrative neural defect that he labels *schizotaxia*.

The imposition of a social learning history on schizotaxic individuals results in a schizotypic personality organization. That is, all schizotaxic individuals obtain a schizotypic personality organization regardless of environmental conditions. Most of these individuals will remain compensated. However, those who encounter certain detrimental influences (e.g., schizophrenogenic mothering) will decompensate into schizophrenics. In light of this model, only a few of those individuals who have inherited the neural defect and are thereby predisposed to schizophrenia, will manifest the disorder.

Despite the wide disparity among theoretical models, most can be classified as elabourate extensions of the nature versus nurture controversy. It is apparent that this debate cannot be adequately resolved until a broader base of knowledge is developed.

Until that time, it may be wise to bear in mind that genetic research does not necessarily negate endeavors supporting contextualist and psychodynamic conceptions. Instead, genetic research addresses both environmental and genetic factors, and is interested in delineating the effects of each separately and in interaction as they pertain to schizophrenia.

HUMAN GENETIC DISORDERS

Thousands of inherited diseases caused by altered genes and chromosomal abnormalities affect humans. These disorders cause problems such as physical deformities, metabolic dysfunction, and developmental problems. Medical surveys indicate that roughly 1 percent of newborns in the United States have a single-gene defect. As many as 1 baby in 200 is born with a chromosomal abnormality serious enough to produce physical defects or mental retardation.

It is misleading to say that a person "inherits the gene" for a disease, since humans are born with the same number and types of genes. We inherit allele forms of specific genes, and these alleles may be defective. Most of the known inherited genetic disorders are caused by the mutation of a single gene, resulting in alleles that produce disease. These defects often produce disturbances in the body's biochemical processes, such as inhibiting the action of an important enzyme or stimulating the overproduction of a harmful substance. Frequently the consequences of such problems can cause severe disability or be fatal.

Many single-gene disorders follow Mendelian patterns of inheritance. A mother and father each pass an allele for a specific gene on to a child. If one of the alleles is defective and causes disease, the child will develop the disease according to a dominant-recessive pattern of inheritance. For example, cystic fibrosis (CF), a metabolic disorder that causes a progressive loss of lung function, is caused by a mutation in the recessive allele of a gene responsible for regulating salt content in the lungs. The recessive allele is unable to direct the production of a key protein, resulting in a salt imbalance that causes thick, suffocating mucus to build up in the lungs. If a baby inherits the defective allele from just one parent, no disease results. But the infant who inherits the defective allele from both parents will be born with the disease.

In other cases, a single dominant allele causes genetic disease. Huntington's disease, a condition characterized by involuntary movements, dementia, and eventually death, is caused by the inheritance of a pair of alleles in which a defective allele dominates the normal allele for the gene. An affected parent has a 50 percent chance of passing the defective allele to a child. A child who inherits the dominant defective allele from just one parent will develop the disease.

Other inherited genetic diseases are caused by defects in the genes found on the X chromosome. Hemophilia, the inability of the blood to clot and heal a wound, is caused by a defect in an allele located on the X chromosome that helps produce proteins involved in the clotting process. Women who inherit this defective allele usually have the normal allele on their second X chromosome, which produces enough of these clotting proteins for the body to remain healthy. Women who inherit this faulty allele have a 50 percent chance of passing the defective allele on to their children. Males who inherit this defective allele do not have a normal version of the allele on their Y chromosome and so cannot produce clotting proteins to heal wounds. Hemophiliacs are almost always males who have inherited an X chromosome with the faulty allele from their mother.

Other genetic disorders arise due to the inheritance of an abnormal number of chromosomes or a defective chromosome structure. These chromosomal abnormalities have a devastating impact: Many fetuses with such defects, particularly those with missing chromosomes, will die prenatally, resulting in miscarriage (spontaneous abortion). In other cases, newborns with chromosomal abnormalities suffer from physical problems or varying degrees of mental retardation. Down syndrome occurs when an individual's cells carry an extra copy of chromosome 21. People born with this condition have characteristic facial features, short stature, severe developmental disabilities, and a shortened life expectancy.

Genetics and Cancer

Cancer is a common name for many diseases that affect different body tissues, including the skin and the liver. All cancers involve alterations in genes that control cell division. These alterations cause cells to replicate abnormally and form tumors. Cancers generally arise from mutations that occur directly in the somatic cells, any cells of the body with the exception of the gametes (sperm and egg cells). Since the genetic mutations have not occurred in gametes, the mutations are not inherited by the next generation.

While cancer is not a traditional inherited genetic disorder, scientists have determined that a genetic component plays a strong role in the development of the disease. Geneticists have identified many different genes with certain alleles that appear to increase an individual's susceptibility to cancer. A notable example involves two genes linked to breast cancer. Researchers estimate that more than half of the women with a family history of breast cancer who inherit mutated alleles of these two genes, known as BRCA1 and BRCA2, will develop breast cancer by the age of 70. In contrast, women who lack either of the mutated alleles have only a 13 percent chance of developing the disease. For many cancers, researchers believe that mutations in several different genes must accumulate before cancer develops. As a person ages, errors in DNA replication may occur during cell division, or cells may be damaged by exposure to certain environmental factors, including cigarette smoke, radiation, and chemical pollutants. As a result, an accumulation of mutations may develop in two types of genes: tumor suppressor genes and oncogenes. Tumor suppressor genes normally function to halt cell division, while oncogenes function to activate cell division. A mutation in either type of gene can stimulate nonstop cell division. These types of defects have been linked to some cases of leukemia as well as to cancers of the ovaries, lungs, colon, and other organs.

Genetics and Aging

A growing area of study focuses on the link between aging and genetics. Scientists have determined that structures called telomeres, long, repetitive sequences of nucleotides at the end of chromosomes, affect the aging process. Each time a cell divides, telomeres become shorter. When the structures shorten to a certain length, the process of cell division terminates. The cells of these chromosomes continue to live, but they never divide again. Laboratory tests suggest that an enzyme produced in gamete cells of the human body, called telomerase, can maintain telomere length in human cells, enabling them to continue dividing, perhaps indefinitely.

Scientists hoping to lasso the life-extending properties of telomerase have been confounded by research indicating that telomerase is also active in rapidly dividing cancer cells. Before telomerase can be used to slow or halt aging, scientists must learn how to manipulate the enzyme so that it does not promote cancer growth.

Genes and Behaviour

Scientists actively explore the links between genes and behaviour to determine both the patterns and the limits of genetic influence. Such studies continue to be controversial because behaviour or mental processes can be difficult to measure objectively. Furthermore, many behavioral traits, both normal and abnormal, are complex, influenced by many genes as well as by personal experiences. Studies of the possible genetic components of psychiatric disorders have yielded mixed results. Geneticists have identified at least two genes linked to schizophrenia, a condition characterized by hallucinations, delusion, paranoia, and other symptoms. Other studies that reported the discovery of genes that influence bipolar disorder (also known as manic-depressive illness) and alcoholism have been reversed or questioned. Though attempts to identify genes linked to these disorders have been flawed, scientists have little doubt that the conditions do have a genetic component.

Scientists have established links between genes and certain antisocial or violent behaviors. For instance, researchers have identified a gene on the X chromosome that has been tied to extremely violent behaviour in men.

They identified the gene in members of several families with a multigenerational history of violent, criminal behaviour. They identified gene codes for monoamine oxidase inhibitor (MAO), an enzyme that helps nerve cells in the brain communicate with each other. Males in an affected family who inherit a defective allele for MAO do not produce enough of the enzyme. As a result, low levels of MAO change the activity of certain brain nerve cells, possibly contributing to socially unacceptable behaviour.

While research suggests that men who have a defective allele for the MAO gene are more prone to aggressive behaviour, experts cite numerous reasons for concern and doubt. Few scientists believe that a single gene could have a leading role in influencing complex behaviors. Others charge that these kinds of investigations promote an unreasonably simplistic view of genetic determinism, in which genes can be blamed for certain behaviors. Critics note that studies have identified many men who carried the defective allele for MAO production and never committed a violent act. Clearly, nongenetic influences—as varied as an individual's family life, work circumstances, attitudes, diet, and emotional state—affect complex behaviors.

IDENTIFYING GENETIC DISORDERS

Health-care professionals who specialize in genetic disorders use a variety of methods to identify inherited conditions. Analysis of a family medical history, known as pedigree analysis, is used to track the transmission of a condition through generations. Blood tests that identify specific DNA sequences can reveal carriers of a disease-causing gene who have no symptoms of the disease.

Geneticists collect a person's medical family history to trace the inheritance of a genetic trait among multiple generations. The information is placed in a pedigree, which resembles a traditional multigenerational family tree but includes information about individuals who were diagnosed with a particular disorder or who suffered from certain medical symptoms. A pedigree can help researchers recognize diseases that express themselves in dominant or recessive alleles. Dominant disorders affect every generation. Recessive disorders may cluster in a single generation, reflecting when two parents who both carry a recessive allele for a disease have one or more children who develop the disease. A pedigree can also identify diseases that show X-linked inheritance.

Pedigree analysis can be useful when combined with certain genetic tests. A blood sample taken from a person who is at risk for a genetic disorder can be compared with a DNA sequence known to cause the disorder in question. Other genetic tests can reveal if a person has extra chromosomes, missing chromosomes, or chromosomes that have attached to one another in unusual ways. In some cases, these chromosomal abnormalities may produce genetic disorders in children or they may affect a person's ability to conceive a child. Genetic testing can also identify disorders in a fetus, enabling parents to learn early in a pregnancy if a fetus will likely be born with health problems or develop them later in life.

Presymptomatic testing can identify DNA abnormalities in a person before health problems develop. In the case of certain inherited heart conditions, for example, these tests enable a person to make healthy lifestyle changes or take other preventative measures, such as medications, to lower the risk of illness or death.

Medical genetic testing raises challenging issues because such tests typically provide statistical possibilities rather than a definite prediction of whether a person will develop a given genetic disease. A test result may indicate, for example, that a person has a 75 percent risk of developing colon cancer by the age of 65. Such results enable a physician to perform appropriate screening tests on the at-risk person in order to identify the disease at its earliest stages, when it is most treatable. At the same time, however, physicians must decide at what age the person's screening should begin and whether the benefits of early screening are worth the drawbacks of frequent screening.

These drawbacks include expense, patient anxiety and discomfort, and exposure to radioactivity or other harmful substances used in testing. Different problems are posed by genetic screening tests that diagnose conditions for which no preventive measures exist, such as Alzheimer's disease, a progressive brain disorder that causes the loss of mental function.

People may find it devastating to learn that they are at risk for a deadly disease that cannot be prevented by medical measures or lifestyle choices.

Gene Therapy

A recent development in genetic technology known as gene therapy focuses on curing inherited disorders. In experiments using gene therapy, researchers have replaced defective genes with normal alleles, inactivated a mutated gene, or inserted a normal form of a gene into a chromosome. The earliest success in human gene therapy involved the treatment of infants who cannot produce adenosine deaminase (ADA), an enzyme important to normal function of the immune system. Scientists have successfully inserted the normal allele for the gene that codes for the enzyme into cells in ADA-deficient children. Preliminary evidence indicates that this gene therapy leads to better immune function in recipients. Researchers are also exploring gene therapy's potential to help treat people with many other conditions, including certain cancers, hemophilia, heart disease, and cystic fibrosis.

Although the United States Food and Drug Administration (FDA) has approved more than 400 clinical trials in gene therapy, this method of treating disease remains far from an unqualified medical success. Treatments usually produce some improvement in the underlying condition, but not enough to consider the therapy suitable for large-scale use. The death of a patient involved in a gene therapy experiment in 1999 caused the National Institutes of Health (NIH), a federal agency that monitors gene therapy studies, to reevaluate the safety and effectiveness of gene therapy clinical trials.

Human Genome Project

The Human Genome Project is the most ambitious project in the history of biology. The program's challenging goal was to identify and sequence all of the DNA in human chromosomes. The project was initiated in 1990 in the United States with government funding, and it rapidly grew into an international consortium of academic centers and drug companies in China, France, Germany, Japan, the United Kingdom, and the United States. The consortium initially hoped to reach its goal by the year 2005.

In 1998 Celera Genomics, a privately funded biotechnology firm, announced that it would sequence the human genome by the year 2000 using different sequencing strategies than those used by the public consortium. This announcement triggered a heated race between Celera Genomics and the public consortium to complete the genome project. In June 2000 both teams declared victory when they jointly announced that they had separately completed a rough draft of the genome. The two teams published their findings simultaneously, although in two different journals, in February 2001. The draft provided a basic outline of 90 percent of the human genome. Scientists from the public consortium completed the final sequencing of the human genome in April 2003, two years earlier than planned.

The completed human genome has provided scientists with a detailed blueprint of our complex genetic code. Large computer databases of genetic information enable scientists to look for patterns and relationships among the actions of different genes. Among the findings about the human genome was that the number of genes in the human genome is much lower than was predicted—only about 20,000 to 25,000 genes compared to the expected 100,000 genes. This number is a little more than twice the number of genes found in the fruit fly.

Scientists are now turning their attention to studying how the relatively low number of genes in the human genome can produce the complex structures found in humans. Scientists have long known that a single gene produces a single protein and that this single protein subsequently may be processed into several different proteins. In a new science known as proteomics, scientists seek to identify and understand the function of all the proteins in the human body. They theorize that there may be many more proteins than there are genes—that is, more than 25,000. Among other advances, the database of proteins derived from proteomics is expected to help scientists better understand the regulation of gene expression in the body and how it leads to the complexity of cellular structures and functions. In addition, proteomics may lead to the development of breakthrough drugs for a variety of genetic disorders.

GENE REGULATION IN EUKARYOTES

Like prokaryotes, eukaryotic organisms do not want to express all of their genes all of the time. Given the complexity of multicellular eukaryotes, gene regulation in these organisms needs to be very complex. This module provides a brief overview of the various levels of regulation of gene expression in eukaryotes, and takes a look at the basics of transcriptional regulation; a detailed look at eukaryotic transcriptional regulation is beyond the scope of this course.

The Need for Gene Regulation in Eukaryotes

Eukaryotes need to regulate their genes for different reasons than prokaryotes. In prokaryotes, gene regulation allowed them to respond to their environment efficiently and economically. While eukaryotes can respond to their environment, the main reason higher eukaryotes need to regulate their genes is cell specialization. Whereas prokaryotes are (relatively speaking) simple, unicellular organisms, multicellular eukaryotes consist of hundreds of different cell types, each differentiated to serve a different specialized function. Each cell type differentiates by activating a different subset of genes. Because of the multitude of cell types, the regulation of gene expression required to bring about such differentiation is necessarily complex. One way this complexity is demonstrated is in multiple levels of regulation of gene expression.

Levels of Regulation

Before we discuss the specifics of regulation, it is necessary to understand that "gene expression" covers the entire process from transcription through protein synthesis. The final measure of whether or not a gene is "expressed" is if the protein is produced, because it is protein that will ultimately carry out the function specified by the gene.

We've seen numerous examples of how eukaryotic cells are more complex than prokaryotic cells. One obvious example of this is the presence of a nucleus in eukaryotic cells, which separates transcription from translation in a way not seen in prokaryotes. Furthermore, eukaryotic transcripts must be processed before they can be translated. Here is a diagram outlining the steps involved in the production of a protein in eukaryotic cells: Regulation can occur at any point in this pathway; specifically, it occurs at the levels of transcription, RNA processing, mRNA lifetime (longevity), and translation. Each of these types of regulation will be considered in turn.

Regulation of RNA Processing

After transcription, the RNA must be processed before it can be translated. As described elsewhere, RNA processing involves addition of a 5' cap, addition of a 3' poly (A) tail, and removal of introns. This processing represents another level of regulation of gene expression, particularly in regard to splicing out of introns.

Regulation can be of two types:
- Whether an RNA gets processed;
- Which exons are retained in the mRNA.

The first type of regulation can determine whether or not an mRNA gets translated. If an RNA is not processed, it will not be transported out of the nucleus, and will not be translated.

The second type of regulation can affect the function of the protein produced. Some genes have exons that can be exchanged in a process known as exon shuffling. For example, a gene with four exons might be spliced differently in two different cell types. In cell 1, exons 1, 2, and 4 would be used in the mRNA:

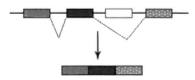

In cell 2 on the other hand, exons 1, 3, and 4 would be used:

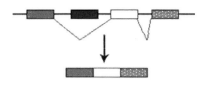

In each of these cases, the polypeptide produced could have a different function. In mammals, for example, the calcitonin gene produces a hormone in one cell type, and a neurotransmitter in another cell type, due to exon shuffling. In *Drosophila*, alternate splicing of the *sex-lethal* RNA can produce an mRNA encoding a functional polypeptide, or one with a premature stop codon that encodes a short, nonfunctional polypeptide.

Regulation of RNA Longevity

Imagine two mRNA molecules: one lasts for five minutes in the cytoplasm before being degraded, while the other one manages to linger for an hour before being degraded. If both are translated continually while they exist, it is obvious that more of the second polypeptide will be produced than the first. This is the principle behind regulation of RNA longevity. mRNAs from different genes have their approximate lifespan encoded in them; this serves to help regulate how much of each polypeptide is produced. The information for lifespan is found in the 3' UTR. The sequence AUUUA, when found in the 3' UTR, is a signal for early degradation (and therefore short lifetime). The more times the sequence is present, the shorter the lifespan of the mRNA. Because it is encoded in the nucleotide sequence, this is a set property of each different mRNA; the longevity of an mRNA can't be varied.

Regulation of Translation

Whether or not an mRNA molecule is translated can be regulated as well. The various mechanisms of translational regulation are incompletely understood, but there are many documented examples (particularly in embryonic development) of mRNA molecules that are present routinely, but are only translated under certain circumstances. For example, many animals sequester large amounts of mRNA in their eggs, and those mRNA molecules are not translated unless the egg is fertilized.

Regulation of Transcription

Whether or not a gene is transcribed is the major way that gene expression is regulated in eukaryotes, as it was in prokaryotes. There are some major differences between transcriptional regulation in prokaryotes and eukaryotes. For one thing, because of the complexity of eukaryotic patterns of gene expression, each eukaryotic gene needs its own promoter. In other words, eukaryotic genes are not organized into operons. Another difference is that prokaryotic genes are regulated primarily by repressors. Although repressors occasionally play a role in eukaryotes, eukaryotic genes are primarily regulated by transcriptional activators. These activators are transcription factors.

Regulatory Elements of Eukaryotic Genes

As discussed in the module on transcription, eukaryotic genes have promoters that are recognized by basal transcription factors (such as TFIID). In addition to the promoter, eukaryotic genes have one or more enhancers. These are DNA sequences associated with the gene being regulated, and whereas the promoter is responsible for initiating low levels of transcription and determining the transcription start site, enhancers are responsible for increasing ("enhancing") transcription levels, and they are responsible for regulating cell- or tissue-specific transcription (i.e. the transcription responsible for differentiation). There are some other basic differences between enhancers and promoters, which are outlined in the module on transcription.

Enhancers function by being recognized and bound to by transcription factors. These are not the basal-type transcription factors (such as TFIID) discussed elsewhere. These are specialized transcription factors, of which there are very many types (all are proteins). A very large number of enhancer elements has been identified and characterized, and each different enhancer has its own transcription factor that it binds to.

Tissue-specific Gene Expression

How is a gene turned on in one cell type, and not in another? It depends primarily on whether the transcription factor for the gene's enhancer is active or not in a cell. To illustrate this, let's consider two different genes - one is regulated by enhancer A, which is recognized by transcription factor A, and the other gene is regulated by enhancer B, which is recognized by transcription factor B. In one cell type (let's say muscle, for the sake of argument), transcription factor A might be active whereas transcription factor B might not. In such a cell, only the first gene would be transcribed:

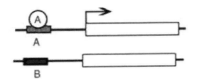

In another cell type (e.g. epidermis), transcription factor B would be active, and transcription factor A would not. In this cell, only the second gene would be transcribed:

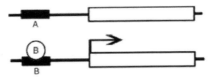

So how is it determined which transcription factors are active in which cell types? The answer to this question is very complicated, and not completely understood. However, there are a number of mechanisms by which transcription factors can be regulated:

- Often, the presence or absence of a transcription factor in a cell is the determining step. If the factor is present, the gene is transcribed. If not, then the gene is not transcribed. The presence of a transcription factor, of course, depends upon the activity of the gene encoding that transcription factor, which forces us to ask how the gene encoding the transcription factor is regulated, which pretty much brings us back to where we began.

- Transcription factors can be activated by environmental signals. For example, virtually all organisms have a set of genes called heat shock genes that encode proteins that help the organism survive heat stress. These genes are activated under conditions of heat stress, under the control of a transcription factor called heat shock transcription factor. This factor is always present, but is only activated when greatly increased temperatures are detected.

- Transcription factors can be activated by signals from other cells in the same organism. Such signals include hormones and growth factors.

Hormones must bind to a specific receptor on the target cell, and the receptor mediates the cellular effects of the signal. There are two basic mechanisms used, one for steroid hormones, and one for peptide hormones:

- Steroid hormones are lipid (actually cholesterol) derivatives, such as testosterone and progesterone. These hormones can cross the cytoplasmic membrane into a cell, where they bind to their specific receptor. Steroid receptors are transcription factors, and when they bind to their ligand, they become activated and initiate transcription of a specific set of genes.
- Peptide hormones cannot cross the cytoplasmic membrane, and so must bind to a receptor on the cell surface. When bound to its ligand, these receptors initiate a series of biochemical reactions inside the cell, with the ultimate result being the activation of a transcription factor (often by phosphorylation of the transcription factor), which initiates transcription of a specific set of genes.

Developmental Genetics

The primary function of the majority of genes in eukaryotic organisms is to coordinate the development of embryos. This module takes a look at some of the basic principles underlying the role of genes in embryonic development. In most of the other modules of this course, the effects of genes are examined with regard to their effect on the phenotype of the juvenile or adult organism. In reality, however, the vast majority of these phenotypes are established during embryonic development, because most genes function to generate the pattern (the 'shape') of the developing embryo.

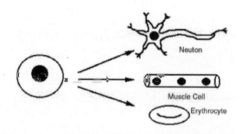

Loss of function of a particular gene results in an abnormality in development, which manifests itself as a phenotype in the adult. In this sense, virtually all of eukaryotic genetics is developmental genetics, even though we haven't considered it as such. The field of developmental biology is concerned with the function of genes in embryogenesis. The central question of developmental biology is the following:

How does a single cell, the fertilized egg (or zygote), manage to produce an extremely complex adult organism, which is composed not only of trillions of cells, but of thousands of different types of cells (such as nerve cells, muscle cells, etc.)?

There is a simple answer to this question, and that is that cells differentiate. In other words, different cells become specialized to carry out different functions by following different developmental pathways. But how does this occur? How do cells know what pathway to follow?

The Mosaic Theory of Development

One early theory (in the late 1890's) that attempted to explain the process of differentiation was the mosaic theory, as outlined by Wilhelm Roux and August Weismann. This theory proposed that there were determinants that specified the various differentiation pathways.

The theory stated that these determinants would all be present in the zygote, but as cell division occurred after fertilization, the determinants would be unequally inherited by the offspring cells. This is known as qualitative cell division. The set of determinants would thus be divided up until each cell contained only one type of determinant, and that determinant would determine the fate of that cell. When Mendel's work was rediscovered in the early 1900's and the concept of the 'gene' was developed, it was believed that the genes were the determinants that were divided up during cell division.

This idea is an appealing one because of its simplicity, but the theory is impeded by one small problem: IT IS WRONG. Evidence was accumulated over sixty years that disproved the notion that genes are divided up in development. The final nail in the coffin of this theory came from nuclear transplantation studies done using amphibians in the early 1960's. In these studies, nuclei were isolated from tadpole intestinal cells (differentiated cells) and injected into eggs that had their own haploid nuclei removed.

A small percentage of the injected eggs developed into completely normal adult frogs! These frogs had developed using only the genetic information found in a tadpole intestinal nucleus. Therefore, a tadpole intestinal nucleus must contain all of the genetic information necessary to allow the differentiation of every cell type in an adult frog. If the mosaic theory were correct, this would not be the case; a tadpole intestinal nucleus would have only the genetic information necessary to cause the differentiation of an intestinal cell.

Note: The frogs produced by this procedure would be genetically identical to the frog from which the intestinal cell nucleus was obtained. In other words, they would be clones. In fact, these experiments comprised the earliest successful cloning of vertebrate organisms. The recent cloning of Dolly the sheep was done for the same reasons as outlined above: demonstrating that differentiated mammalian nuclei (from mammary gland in this case) have all of the genetic information necessary to drive the development of a normal adult organism.

The Theory of Differential Gene Expression

If all nuclei in an organism contain the same genetic information (as we know they do), then how does differentiation occur? The explanation for this is found in the Theory of Differential Gene Expression. This theory states that differentiation occurs as a result of expression in a particular cell of only a subset of the total genes present. For example, if a cell expresses only the set of genes that causes muscle differentiation, then that cell will differentiate into a muscle cell. Alternatively, if the cell expresses only the set of genes that causes spleen cell differentiation, then the cell will differentiate into a spleen cell. This is a fairly simple concept, but it hasn't really answered the question. The question has now become: how do cells activate only a certain set of genes (inactivating all other genes), and how do they know which set of genes to activate?

The answer to this question is fairly straightforward as well: the set of genes activated in a cell is dependent on the set of transcription factors found in the cell. Using the muscle cell example from above, the cell activates the muscle-specific genes because it contains transcription factors that specifically activate the muscle-specific genes.

If you think about this for a minute, you'll realise that we still haven't answered the question; we've only changed it again. Now the question becomes: how did the cell come to contain only that specific set of transcription factors? Well, those transcription factors are encoded by genes, and those genes are regulated by other specific transcription factors. Those transcription factors are in turn encoded by other genes, which are regulated by still other transcription factors, etc. As you can see, there is a hierarchy of genes within each cell.

Genes are expressed that encode transcription factors, which activate other genes that encode transcription factors, which activate other genes that bring about differentiation along a specific pathway. How many levels are there to the hierarchy? From what we've seen so far, the hierarchy seems to go on forever. Each set of transcription factors is encoded by genes that are activated by yet another set of transcription factors. It must end somewhere, but where?

Master Control Genes

In one sense, it ends with master control genes. A master control gene is the first gene activated in a hierarchy that leads to differentiation along a particular pathway. Master control genes encode the first transcription factor in a hierarchy; a master control gene product activates the next set of genes that encodes the next set of transcription factors, and the cascade of gene expression has been set in motion.

Let's look again at the muscle cell example considered earlier. The master control 'gene' for muscle development is actually a family of genes called the MyoD gene family. These genes encode HLH-type transcription factors. How do we know these are the master control genes for muscle? Master control genes have a particular property. Because they initiate muscle differentiation, if the MyoD genes are activated in other cell types, they cause those cells to transdifferentiate into muscle. For example, hepatocytes (liver cells) or adipocytes (fat cells) that are caused to express the MyoD genes (using tricks of molecular biology) will change from their normal phenotype into muscle cells.

So how are the master control genes regulated? There are two basic ways that this can happen. One way is through the process of induction. Induction occurs when once cell sends a signal to another cell, telling it to differentiate a certain way. The signal, usually a diffusable protein, causes the recipient cell to activate the appropriate master control gene product. This is how muscle differentiation occurs. Signals from other cells cause the MyoD genes to become active in the cells receiving the signal, and muscle differentiation is initiated.

GENETIC CODE

The role of the cytoplasm, however, differs from that of the chromosomal materials in the following respects. Different germ cells differ effectively in their genes, and it is to these gene differences that the appearance of diverse characteristics in different individuals is due. But as a rule there is no evidence that the cytoplasm of different germ cells is effectively diverse in such a way as to produce different characteristics in different individuals. It is therefore the former the chromosomes with their genes that are commonly classified as the 'materials of heredity' more properly perhaps the 'materials of hereditary diversity'. The cytoplasm might correspondingly be called the 'materials of bodily differentiation.

Following the prevailing usage therefore, we may define the genetic system or material of heredity as follows: The genetic system consists of those parts of the cells that are effectively diverse in different germ cells, these diversities causing different characteristics to appear in the different individuals produced.

In rare cases, in certain plants, it is found that the cytoplasm contains programmes bodies which may differ in different germ cells and so cause differences in the characteristics of the individuals developed from them. In such cases the cytoplasm, or at least the programmes bodies it contains, must be included as part of the genetic system. But in most organisms the genetic system consists of the chromosomes with their genes.

Constitution of the Chromosomes The Groups of Characters Linkage

Each of the chromosomes (save in some cases the Y-chromosome) is composed, as we have seen, of many diverse genes. In the wild, unmodified individuals, in the fruit-fly, the genes are such as produce the 'normal' or 'wild-type' characteristics of the individuals. The genes of any chromosome become modified in the course of time, in the process known as mutation.

The modified genes produce altered characteristics, most of which are recessive, while the normal characteristics, when mated to the modified characteristics, are dominant. A few of the modified characteristics, however, are dominant when mated with the normal or wildtype characters. The modified characteristics resulting from mutation are in most, if not all, cases defects, as compared with the normal characters. Thus the normal, dominant characters form a standard condition, of which the defective and recessive mutated characters are modifications.

The diverse genes of any chromosome are designated, so far as they have received names, by the name of one of the modified characters which it helps to produce. Thus the gene yellow, near the upper or left end of the X-chromosome of Drosophila, produces in its mutated condition the modified body programmes yellow; while in its unmodified condition it produces the normal grey programmes of the wild fly. In the maps of all the names apply to the modified or mutated condition of the gene.

For every such modified gene there is a corresponding unmodified normal or wild-type gene. It is the custom to designate the wild-type gene from which any modified gene is derived by writing with the name or abbreviation for the modified gene the sign +. Thus yellow + or y + or + y signifies the normal wild-type gene that produces grey body programmes; white + or w + signifies the normal gene located at I, i .5, which produces red eyes in place of white ones. The genes of any one of the chromosomes, as X, or a given autosome, become modified in many different ways, so that different examples of the same chromosome have different sets of genes.

The diversity of genes in the chromosomes of different germ cells causes diversities in development, with resulting different characteristics in the individuals produced. The characteristics produced by the action of the genes of any chromosome follow in the individuals of successive generations the distribution to the offspring of the genes that produce them. Thus many characteristics follow the course of the X-chromosome; many follow each autosome; a few may follow the Y-chromosome.

Since a large group of characteristics follows each chromosome, the result is that characteristics pass from parent to offspring in groups. As an X-chromosome passes from the father into his daughters, all the genes, and all the characteristics that they produce, pass together into the daughters. Here, of course, some of the recessive characteristics may remain hidden in the presence of dominant genes in the second X- chromosome carried by the daughters.

But all may reappear anew when in a later generation this X-chromosome is again by itself in a male. Except in so far as there is exchange or crossing-over with the other chromosome of the pair, all the characteristics that depend on the genes of a particular chromosome pass together into the individual that receives that chromosome, and this continues for generation after generation.

Thus, in Drosophila, suppose that a male has white eyes and yellow body, two characteristics connected with genes in the single X-chromosome. He is mated with a female that has red eyes and grey body, again owing to genes in the X-chromosome. In the daughters of these two, the two types of X-chromosomes are present together. These daughters produce offspring in a third generation. Some of their sons receive the X-chromosome that came from the original male; these will have white eyes and yellow body. Other sons receive the X-chromosome that came from the original female; these have red eyes and grey body. Only a very minute proportion of the offspring have the reverse combinations of characteristics white eyes with grey body, and red eyes with yellow body.

The two characters originally together white and yellow appear to be linked, and the same is true of the other combination, red and grey. The original combinations do not readily separate.This linkage of characters in heredity was observed before it was known that characteristics depend on chromosomes.

Many theories were invented to account for it, until it was discovered that it is due to the fact that the linked characters depend on genes that are in the same chromosome. All characteristics that depend on the same chromosome form what is called a linkage group. Since there are different numbers of chromosomes in different organisms, there are correspondingly different numbers also of linkage groups.

These linkage groups are of great importance in heredity. They reveal to us many things about the nature and action of the genetic system. We shall therefore examine these groups in a typical organism, selecting for this purpose the animal in which they are best known, namely, Drosophila melanogaster.

The Groups of Linked Characters in Drosophila

The fruit-fly has, as we have seen, four pairs of chromosomes. On the genes in these four pairs of chromossomes depend several hundred known inherited characteristics. These many characteristics form four linked groups, according to their dependence on genes in the X-chromo- some, or in the chromosomes II, III or IV. It is to be noted that all of the characteristics that depend on genes in either one of a given pair of chromosomes constitute a single linkage group, since all those characteristics may become connected with the genes of a single one of the chromosomes. Thus the number of linkage groups is the same as the number of pairs of chromosomes. In the course of breeding successive generations, linkage of charact-eristics shows itself in the fact that certain characteristics (dependent on genes in the same chromosome), which are present together in one parent, are present together also in the individual descendants.

This is best seen on comparing grandchildren with grandparents. In this case one grandparent had the combination white-yellow, the other the combination red-grey. The same two combinations reappear in the grandchildren. In addition there are a very few 'cross-overs', having the new combinations white-grey in some individuals, red-yellow in others.

But almost all the grandchildren get both the characteristics from the same gandparent. If the original grandparents have the other combinations, grey-white and yellow-red, then the majority of the grandchildren show these combinations. Thus just what combination of characteristics the individual grandchildren have depends on what characteristics were united in the grandparents. But this is the case of course only for characteristics whose genes lie in the same chromosome. If two characteristics depend on genes that are in different pairs of chromosomes, then the combinations that were present in the grandparents are no more frequent in the descendants than are the reverse combinations.

It is in many respects most convenient to think of linkage in terms of the gametes. The combination of genes that are present in the gametes can often be determined by examination of the offspring produced. With relation to the gametes, linkage can be characterized as follows. When an individual (zygote) is formed by the union of two gametes, each bearing in one of its chromosomes a certain combination of linked genes, this same individual later produces gametes of which

the majority have these same combinations of linked genes. Often also there is a minority of gametes that have the genes combined in a new way, as a result of crossing-over. In the fruit-fly, crossing-over occurs only in the females, not in the males.

Thus if a male individual is formed by the union of two gametes carrying certain combinations of linked genes, then later such a male produces only gametes having the same combinations of linked genes. This fact is extremely convenient for determining what characteristics are linked in Drosophila.There are many other organisms in which crossingover is not limited to one sex. By breeding for successive generations and by the study of exchanges between the chromosomes, the following groups of linked characters have been found in the fruit-fly.

Group IA large group of sex-linked characters, more than 100 in number.These all follow in heredity the distribution of X-chromosomes, as described in earlier pages. Any two or more of these characters may be linked together and connected with the same X-chromosome.

Group IIA large group of typical Mendelian characters, 50 to 100 or more in number. These follow the method of distribution of autosomes, and any two or more of the group may be connected with the same autosome.

Group III.Another large group of typical Mendelian characters, 50 to 100 or more in number, following the method of distribution of autosomes. Any two or more of this group may be connected with the same autosome, but a character of Group III is not linked with any character of Group II.

Group IV.A small group of typical Mendelian characters, only 5 or 6 known.These are not linked with any of the characters of Groups I, II or III.All of the 300 or more characters known in this species fall into one or the other of these four groups. The nature of the characters found in the different groups is considered on later pages.

Thus here the number of linked groups is the same as the number of pairs of chromosomes. There are three large groups and one very small one; likewise there are three large pairs of chromosomes and one very small pair. It is natural to conclude, therefore, that the groups of linked characters correspond to the pairs of chromosomes, and that the characteristics in each group are connected with some particular pair. As it turns out, there is conclusive evidence that this is true. The evidence for each of the groups may be summarized as follows:

All the characters in Group I are sex-linked; that is, they follow exactly the distribution of the X-chromosomes. Any character in this group follows a particular X-chromosome and its descendants, wherever that chromosome goes. The characteristics in Group I are thus certainly dependent on genes in the X-chromosomes. The small group of characters known as Group IV has been proved to be connected with the small chromosomes of pair IV. This has been demonstrated in the following manner. By non-disjunction of this fourth pair of chromosomes, some individuals are produced having but one small chromosome (IV). That this is the situation can be seen under the microscope, in properly prepared material.

These individuals with but one of the small chromosomes have the dominant normal or 'wild' characteristics. Such individuals are mated with individuals containing one of the recessive characters of Group IV. One of these recessive characters is 'bent wings'; another is 'eyeless' the individual having no eyes.

Half of the germ cells from the individuals that have but one of the fourth chromosomes are without this chromosome, while half of them have it. These two kinds each unite with germ cells carrying the recessive character 'bent', or 'eyeless'. There are thus produced individuals, half of which have but one of the fourth chromosomes, while the other half have two. In those which contain two, all the characteristics are of the dominant normal type; the recessive character bent or eyeless is not manifested. But in the individuals having but one fourth chromosome, the recessive character is manifested: the individual shows bent wings, or is eyeless. This demonstrates that the characteristics of Group IV are connected with the small chromosomes.

Thus the large linkage Groups II and III are left for the two large V-shaped chromosome pairs, II and III. These chromosomes can be broken into two or more pieces by subjecting them to radiations. When this is done, the characters of the corresponding linkage groups are no longer linked together.Thus in Group III the two genes scarlet and sooty are linked (completely in the male). But when the corresponding large chromosome (III) is broken into two pieces, scarlet and sooty are no longer linked; they may pass to different offspring.

They are evidently connected with the two separated pieces of chromosome III. In the same way the other large chromosome (II) may be broken, and this causes the characteristics of the linkage Group II to separate into two groups. Minute study shows that the chromosomes II and III differ a little, in size and form, so that with practice it becomes possible to distinguish one from the other under the microscope.

Thus it is proved that each of the four linkage groups is connected with one of the four chromosome pairs; the four groups correspond to the four chromosomes.

In a number of other organisms the number of linked groups of characters has been determined, and also the number of pairs of chromosomes. In every case in which this has been fully worked out, the number of linked groups is the same as the number of pairs of chromosomes. The numbers of groups and of pairs in certain organisms are as follows:

Drosophila melanogaster 4, Drosophila virilis 6, garden pea 8, sweet pea 8, maize10. In man there are twenty-four pairs of chromosomes, including the X's. It is to be expected therefore that there will be found 24 groups of linked characters, one group sex-linked, the other 23 groups typical Mendelian, in their inheritance. But it will be a very long time before these 24 groups are identified.

DIAGNOSIS

Another research difficulty related to that of schizophrenic heterogeneity pertains to clinical diagnosis. The new DSM-III allows for considerable heterogeneity as to who will be diagnosed schizophrenic; persons need to fulfill only a certain number of criteria out of a standard set of possibilities in order to receive the diagnosis.

Schizophrenia cannot be diagnosed unless signs of the disorder have been present for at least 6 months. Illnesses of shorter duration, or illnesses that have resulted in the face of a psychosocial stressor and appear to be transient in nature are no longer included.

In fact, these disorders are not even considered to be subtypes of schizophrenia. These changes in diagnostic criteria have left schizophrenia researchers in a peculiar bind since they now must try to define the onset of a schizophrenic disorder. In the past, the onset of schizophrenia was demarcated by the appearance of psychotic symptoms. However, it is well known that the onset of schizophrenia is often quite insidious, and that prodromal features commonly predate psychotic symptoms.

Logically, it would be best if we could define onset as the point in time when one could predict with virtual certainty that a schizophrenic psychosis would occur. Unfortunately, we still lack the necessary knowledge to make such a prediction, and the definition of onset remains strictly arbitrary. Consequently, the conceptual problem of trying to determine criteria for delineating signs along a continuum marking transitions from a schizophrenia-prone personality structure to a prodomal syndrome to a full-blown psychosis still exists.

Because of these diagnostic difficulties, a standard definition for what constitutes schizophrenia remains to be determined. The absence of a standard definition remains a major hindrance to the progression of this field. The severity of the problem is due to the fact that every research project must of necessity concern itself with identifying those people who have the disorder.

Therefore, the homogeneity of the sample studied and the rigor of the investigation carried out on the sample depend on the accuracy of the diagnosis. Unfortunately, there is no independent validation and only moderate reliability for diagnosing a schizophrenic disorder. Even the combination of moderate interrater reliability and independent validation appears to be inadequate. Consequently, there is no truly homogeneous sample in schizophrenia research. Instead, investigators are forced to contend with the heterogeneous groupings that fit the schizophrenic label, the abundance of contradictory data, and the numerous disagreements over research findings. As long as this state of affairs exists, studies are limited to statistical rather than clinical significance.

At present, many diagnostic difficulties result because little is known about the unity or diversity of schizophrenia. In order to gain a clearer understanding of the nature of the disorder, many investigations have been conducted to determine the degree to which the range of phenotypic expression in schizophrenia is paralleled by genetic heterogeneity. These included certain studies that were designed to investigate whether these subtypes were fundamentally alike or different.

One such study by Winokur, Morrison, Clancy, and Crowe found that hebephrenic probands had more than three times as many schizophrenic relatives as paranoid probands. These authors determined that both children and other secondary cases of schizophrenia in the families of hebephrenics were more likely to be diagnosed hebephrenic as opposed to paranoid schizophrenic. The same type of pattern was established for paranoid schizophrenics.

The children and other secondary cases of schizophrenia in the paranoid probands were more likely to manifest paranoid rather than hebephrenic symptoms. These familial data led the au thors to conclude that process schizophrenia is not likely to be a unitary illness. Instead, they postulated the existence of two types of schizophrenia in the population studied, one of which may manifest itself mostly as hebephrenia but also occasionally as paranoid schizophrenia.

The second type would manifest itself exclusively as paranoid schizophrenia in which there are relatively few schizophrenic relatives. Together, these findings suggest that there may be only one type of hebephrenic schizophrenia, but two types of paranoid schizophrenia, one related genetically to the hebephrenic subtype.

Another study by Kety et al. in 1975 demonstrated that the diagnoses of chronic, latent or borderline, and uncertain schizophrenia tend to cluster in the biological relatives of schizophrenic adoptees. Similarly, a study by Slater and Cowie examined the classical pre-Kraepelinian categories and found a significant association between schizophrenic probands and their schizophrenic offspring with respect to type of category.

Kringlen in 1968 corroborated these results and also demonstrated that the entire set of Kraepelinian subtypes is represented in the children of every type of schizophrenic proband.

These studies are typical of investigations in this area. Their results seem to indicate that some groups of disorders are genetically related, whereas the relationships among others remain unclear. Despite some contradictory findings, the most common results from these studies provide evidence for a common genetic basis among various forms of schizophrenic disorders.

In general, the findings indicate that cases of all subtypes occur in the families of each schizophrenic subtype. They also suggest that only a modest tendency toward subtype resemblance exists within families.

In addition to considering the unity or diversity of schizophrenia, one must also consider the relationship between schizophrenia and other psychiatric disturbances when making clinical diagnoses. This is especially important if one wants to formulate diagnostic criteria that are successful at differentiating among various psychoses.

At present little is known about the specificity of the schizophrenic disorder. However, there is some evidence suggesting a genetic relationship between schizophrenia and other psychiatric disorders. In a study by Reed, Hartley, Anderson, Phillips, and Johnson, a high risk of psychoses for the siblings of psychotics was found.

When the investigators looked at specific disorders, they discovered that the risk for first degree relatives of affective probands to develop a similar disorder was less than their risk of becoming schizophrenic. There is also some indication that the risk of schizophrenia for the offspring of paranoid and hebephrenic schizophrenics is lower than the risk for children of manic—depressives. Even some of the very earliest studies discovered that schizophrenic and affectively ill individuals were about equally prevalent in the families of schizophrenics. Today as well, despite efforts to select clinically homoge neous probands, the occurrence of different types of psychoses in the same family is difficult to avoid.

The suggestion that there may be a similar genetic basis to schizophrenia and other forms of psychoses raises the possibility of overlap in the symptomatology of various psychiatric disturbances; and indeed, this has been found to be the case. Another problem exists in the possibility that symptomatology is not directly related to genetic inheritance. Bleuler speculated that secondary symptoms such as delusions and hallucinations are not inherited. He also suggested that the primary symptoms do not correspond to the transmitted anomaly itself.

As a result of these possibilies, there are some major difficulties involved in basing diagnostic criteria on clinical symptoms. However, there are now some indications that future diagnostic categories will be based on biochemical indicators rather than Behavioural symptoms in order to decrease the heterogeneity of individuals in specified subgroups of psychopathology.

Using biological markers could be advantageous in several ways. First, it could avoid the genetically heterogeneous diagnostic groupings based on standard methods of symptom classification. It is well known that even relatively well formulated clinical subtypes of schizophrenia present diverse symptomatology.

As a result, it is impossible to differentiate between genotypic and phenotypic variations under the present diagnostic systems. The use of biologically independent variables in formulating diagnoses may promote the detection of biological etiologies and the formation of more homogeneous psychiatric diagnostic categories. Individuals who exhibit divergent or less severe clinical symptoms and are thereby excluded from present investigations could be included if they met a biological criterion.

This in turn would allow the high risk population (those individuals with the salient factor) to be identified and studied. The use of a biologically based strategy would also permit the study of non hospitalized and unmedicated individuals, thereby avoiding the inclusion of these confounds within investigations.

In addition to developing biologically based criteria, many other efforts are being made to improve the diagnostic system. For example, the United States— United Kingdom Diagnostic Project, the International Pilot Study of Schizophrenia, and the World Health Organization have provided standardized input on patients for formulating diagnoses, experts to address diagnostic issues, and cross national reference points in order to establish criteria that will improve the reliability and validity of the diagnosis of schizophrenia on an international basis.

Additional reasons for optimism stem from the new trends in schizophrenia nosology. These include an increased reliance on affective symptoms as diagnostically useful, as well as a shift toward incorporating the schizo affective disorders within the affective diagnoses. In addition, the broad use of the schizophrenic label seems to be decreasing as a function of less emphasis being placed on classic schizophrenic symptoms, and more effort being devoted to the use of operationally defined criteria tested for reliability.

Although at present it is still difficult to reach clear and definite conclusions in research dealing with schizophrenia because of the many diagnostic difficulties associated with this disorder, the increasing refinement of diagnostic issues and the development of more sophisticated research techniques makes it possible to conceive of removing the current obstacles to gathering clinically significant data and conducting therapeutic— preventive research.

FAMILY STUDIES

Despite the numerous conceptual and diagnostic difficulties inherent in schizophrenia research, much evidence has been gathered to substantiate the existence of genetic components in the transmission of the disorder. The idea that various forms of mental illness are heritable has existed for many centuries. However, it was not until early in this century that researchers were able to provide actual documentation of this fact.

The first consanguinity study that found a significant increase in the prevalence rate of schizophrenia among relatives of index cases in comparison to the rate of the general population. More specifically, he discovered an age corrected risk for schizophrenia of 4.48per cent and 4.12per cent for other psychoses in the siblings of schizophrenics whose parents were unaffected.

Many other studies have confirmed Rudin's basic finding of a higher rate of schizophrenia in the relatives of samples of schizophrenics than in the samples from the general population. From these studies the rate of schizophrenia in the general population has been calculated to range from.35 to 2.85per cent, with a mean around.85per cent.

The findings from the consanguinity studies also reveal a clear correlation between the degree of blood relationship in relatives of an individual affected with schizophrenia and the risk of those relatives for becoming schizophrenic. More specifically, those relatives who share fewer genes in common with an affected individual show a lower expectancy rate for the disorder than those who share more genes.

In addition, these studies have demonstrated that there are no significant differences between prevalence rates for siblings and other first degree relatives. Although the difference found in the rate of schizophrenia between parents (5.5 per cent) and siblings and children of schizophrenic probands (10.2per cent and 13.9per cent respectively) appears to be large and therefore contradictory to the foregoing statement, this difference has been explained by the fact that these parents are largely selected for a degree of mental health through having been married and having children.

When a correction is made for this factor, the risk in parents of schizophrenics becomes close to that of siblings and children. The somewhat higher risk in children than in siblings of schizophrenics is thought to be due to sampling error. Additional evidence for a genetic factor in the transmission of schizophrenia is found by comparing the different rates of prevalence for the disease among offspring of matings of various psychotic combinations of parents. Estimates have been obtained indicating that the risk for schizophrenia increases as the genetic loading increases. The best estimate of the risk of schizophrenia in the sibling of a schizophrenic is 9.7per cent when neither parent has the disorder. This risk increases to 17.2per cent for the siblings of the proband when one parent also has schizophrenia. When both parents are schizophrenic, the risk to their children ranges between 36.6per cent and 46.3 per cent. Although it can be argued that this raise in risk from 17.2per cent to 46.3per cent for the siblings of a schizophrenic may be due to the extreme environmental conditions created by the mating of two schizophrenics, a study by Kallman reported that a comparable disturbed setting created by the mating of a schizophrenic and a psychopath yielded a sibling risk for schizophrenia of only 15per cent in Gottesman and Shields. The basic findings of these studies have been further substantiated by the results of more recent investigations. For example, a study by Reed et al. reported that the risk to the offspring when neither parent was psychotic increased relative to the number of aunts and uncles who were psychiatrically disturbed.

The difference among estimates of risk is a fact significant for genetic theories. Not only does this difference demonstrate that the risk of mental illness increases as a function of increased genetic loading, but the large amount of variation in the offspring undermines the prediction of environmental theories that virtually all children from dual matings of schizophrenics would be emotionally disturbed.

Another line of evidence for the role of genetic factors in schizophrenia was provided by Manfred Bleuler, who applied the methodology of consanguinity studies to clinical symptomatology and course over time. He discovered that the biological relatives of schizophrenics who also had the disorder tended to have similar ages of onset, presenting clinical pictures, lengths of duration of illness, and outcomes. These findings can be interpreted in either an environmental or genetic fashion. However, a genetic explanation appears to carry more weight because many of the relatives in the study were geographically separated and in some cases did not even know each other. Therefore, the findings of the study indicate that genetic factors play a role in several clinical parametres of schizophrenia.

Although these family studies have contributed much toward the understanding of schizophrenia and have pointed to the role of genetic factors in the development of this disorder, some major difficulties are inherent in their methodology. The earliest family studies did not question the assumption that schizophrenia is heritable and therefore failed to consider the possibility that environmental factors such as family interactions also contribute to the etiology of the disorder.

As a result, these studies provided sources of data on the empirical risk of the occurrence of schizophrenia in different kinds of relatives, but did not elucidate the specific etiology involved in creating those risks. In other words, these studies could indicate if a trait ran in families, but could not specify what aspect of the family determined the trait. Obviously, families share more than genetic similarity, they also share a variety of social, psychological, and cultural experiences. Consequently, the results of these studies can just as validly be interpreted as supporting an environmental position.

Recently, some studies taking an environmental approach have investigated family interactions on the premise that certain conditions of family life can predispose an individual to schizophrenia. The majority of these investigations have focused on deviant role relationships and disordered communication processes among family members.

The findings of these studies generally indicate that deficits in family communication are highly correlated with schizophrenia and high risks for schizophrenia in offspring. In addition, there are some indications that families of schizophrenics contain poorly articulated and rigid role structures in the areas of dominance, autonomy, and sexuality. Despite the success of this type of research, it is unable to establish the occurrence of schizophrenia as a strictly environmental outcome.

In fact, the evidence that is presently available tends to suggest that both genetics and family process play a role in the development of schizophrenia. In light of this evidence, the current mode of investigation has changed to incorporate biological, genetic, psychological, and social factors in the context of complex, multifactorial models of causation when approaching family variables in relation to schizophrenia.

TWIN STUDIES

It was not until the advent of twin studies that the role of genetic and environmental factors in schizophrenia could be more clearly defined. The power of the twin method resides in the environmental similarities and genetic differences between monozygotic and dizygotic twins. Both types of twins share the same intrauterine environment simultaneously with their co-twin. However, monozygotic twins share the same fertilized ovum initially, whereas dizygotic twins are no more genetically alike than ordinary siblings. As a result, one can assume the presence of a genetic factor in determining a trait if the concordance rate for that particular trait is significantly higher for monozygotic as opposed to dizygotic twins.

The methodology of twin studies also provides certain advantages. For example, through the comparison of intrapair resemblance, it becomes possible to identify subtypes or components of schizophrenia that may be more under genetic or environmental control than others. Also, by noting the variability of abnormal personality traits in the monozygotic co-twins of typical schizophrenics, it becomes feasible to identify schizophrenic "equivalents" or schizotypes.

The comparison of monozygotic twins who differ in outcome will permit the formulation of inference about the relationship between life experiences and outcome. It must be kept in mind that the twin study method relies on certain assumptions. These specify that monozygotic twins as such are not specifically predisposed to schizophrenia, and that the environments of monozygotic twins are not systematically more similar than those of dizygotic twins in such a way as to foster the disorder.

Also, when assessing the outcome of these studies it is important to be aware of the usage of statistical age corrections and their effects on research findings. Age corrections incorporate estimates of a lifetime risk for developing schizophrenia in order to compensate for a current sample while the disorder exhibits a variable age of onset. Although several methods have been developed, none is entirely satisfactory, and all present only varying degrees of approximation to the true concordance rate.

It is essential to realise that the absolute size of the concordance rate is not predictive of the relative importance of the genetic contribution to the trait in question. Concordance rates can be expressed in several fashions. The basic difference in methods depends on whether concordance is expressed in terms of the pair or the individual.

The casewise or proband method refers to the proportion of cases with an affected partner, whereas the pairwise rate considers the proportion of pairs in which both twins are affected. The individual or proband concordance method yields a higher per centage than a pairwise concordance. Therefore, only those studies that use the same method are comparable.

The most influential early twin studies were conducted by Kallman and Slater. Even though the two studies contained important differences and suffered from methodological problems, both found a significantly higher concordance rate for schizophrenia among monozygotic twins.

By the end of Kallman's study and with some diagnostic revision, but without statistical age correction, 59per cent of 174 monozygotic pairs and 9per cent of 517 dizygotic pairs were concordant for what Kallman labeled "definite schizophrenia." In Slater's study, 65per cent of 37 monozygotic pairs and 14per cent of 58 same sexed dizygotic pairs were found to be concordant. Both studies used the pairwise method for calculating the concordance rates.

Findings from other earlier studies were basically consistent with these results.

More recently, several studies have been conducted that are methodologically powerful, and that provide highly significant results. One of these studies, reported by Tienari, was conducted on an exclusively male sample in Finland. Initially, this investigator found a zero concordance rate for monozygotic twins.

However, by 1976 the pairwise concordance rate for the sample had risen to 16 per cent. The use of the proband method, the concordance rate for the sample was found to be between 35per cent and 53per cent depending upon which borderline cases were included. As a result, even though it took some time, a significant monozygotic—dizygotic difference was demonstrated.

A study by Kringlen was conducted in Norway and included both male and female twins. His study was especially important for several reasons. His sample was well constructed and contained the largest number of psychotic twins personally investigated among the more recent studies. His investigation was very comprehensive and included case history, pedigree, clinical analysis, rating scale data, and all functional psychoses in addition to schizophrenia. Using the more conservative pairwise method, Kringlen found a significant difference between monozygotic and dizygotic twins with concordance rates ranging from 60per cent for monozygotic probands rated as severe to 25per cent for the most benign.

His results indicated no difference between the concordance rates of monozygotic twins as a function of gender. He reported that whether the sexes of the dizygotic twins were the same or different, the concordance rates did not differ, but were equal to those found in ordinary siblings. These results counter findings from some earlier studies and undermine the psychodynamic thesis that concordance for schizophrenia will increase without regard to genetic similarity, but relative to the amount of likeness and resulting identity confusion among siblings. The findings of another important twin study were reported by Fischer, Harvald, and Hauge in 1969. This study was conducted in Denmark upon a sample that was very representative with respect to twin types and sexes of probands. Only those probands who met strict criteria for chronic or process schizophrenia were included.

Even so, schizophreniform, paranoid, and atypical psychoses in co-twins led to data analysis for quantitative concordance for other than process schizophrenia. As a result of this study, Fischer et al. discovered a pairwise concordance rate of 24per cent for monozygotic twins and 10per cent for dizygotic twins.

In addition, the authors calculated the rates according to the proband method and obtained a 36per cent concordance rate for monozygotic and 18per cent concordance rate for dizygotic pairs. When those co-twins who exhibited a form of schizophrenic disorder different from process schizophrenia were included in their calculations, the investigators obtained proband concordance rates of 56per cent and 26per cent for monozygotic and dizygotic twins respectively.

These figures appear to be good approximations of the true incidence rate, as the twins used in this study were followed long enough to virtually eliminate the need for any statistical age correction.

Fisher went on to report that monozygotic twin pairs concordant for schizophrenia were not at an increased risk for the disorder when compared to discordant monozygotic twins. She did not discover a relationship between severity of disturbance in the proband and the risk of developing psychosis in the co-twin.

The offspring of concordant twins were not at an increased risk for schizophrenia when compared to the offspring of discordant twins. In addition, the likelihood of a discordant twin member producing a schizophrenic child was equal to that of the schizophrenic member of the twin pair. These findings point toward a genetic hypothesis and indicate that the genetic transmission of schizophrenia is not always manifested directly.

The Maudsley Hospital based study of Gottesman and Shields conducted in England obtained similar results to those of the studies reported earlier. These investigators also obtained a significantly increased monozygotic concordance rate over that found in dizygotic twins. Similarly, Pollin, Allen, Hoffer, Stabenau, and Hrubec, in a study based on an American sample, found a higher concordance rate for monozygotic as opposed to dizygotic twins. More specifically, the concordance rate for schizophrenia in monozygotic twins was found to be 3.3 times greater than the rate in dizygotic twins.

7

Microbial Genetics Recombination

Microorganisms have the ability to acquire genes and thereby undergo the process of recombination. In recombination, a new chromosome with a genotype different from that of the parent results from the combination of genetic material from two organisms.

This new arrangement of genes is usually accompanied by new chemical or physical properties. In microorganisms, several kinds of recombination are known to occur.

The most common form is general recombination, which usually involves a reciprocal exchange of DNA between a pair of DNA sequences. It occurs anywhere on the microbial chromosome and is typified by the exchanges occurring in bacterial transformation, bacterial recombination, and bacterial transduction. A second type of recombination, called site-specific recombination, involves the integration of a viral genome into the bacterial chromosome.

A third type is replicative recombination, which is due to the movement of genetic elements as they switch position from one place on the chromosome to another. The principles of recombination apply to prokaryotic microorganisms but not to eukaryotic microorganisms. Eukaryotes exhibit a complete sexual life cycle, including meiosis. In this process, new combinations of a particular gene form during the process of crossing over. This process occurs between homologous chromosomes and is not seen in bacteria, where only a single chromosome exists. Much of the work in microbial genetics has been performed with bacteria, and the unique features of microbial genetics are usually those associated with prokaryotes such as bacteria.

GENETIC RECOMBINATION

A DNA helix usually does not interact with other segments of DNA, and in human cells the different chromosomes even occupy separate areas in the nucleus called "chromosome territories". This physical separation of different chromosomes is important for the ability of DNA to function as a stable repository for information, as one of the few times chromosomes interact is during chromosomal crossover when they recombine.

Chromosomal crossover is when two DNA helices break, swap a section and then rejoin. Recombination allows chromosomes to exchange genetic information and produces new combinations of genes, which increases the efficiency of natural selection and can be important in the rapid evolution of new proteins. Genetic recombination can also be involved in DNA repair, particularly in the cell's response to double-strand breaks.

The most common form of chromosomal crossover is homologous recombination, where the two chromosomes involved share very similar sequences. Non-homologous recombination can be damaging to cells, as it can produce chromosomal translocations and genetic abnormalities. The recombination reaction is catalyzed by enzymes known as recombinases, such as RAD51.

The first step in recombination is a double-stranded break either caused by an endonuclease or damage to the DNA. A series of steps catalyzed in part by the recombinase then leads to joining of the two helices by at least one Holliday junction, in which a segment of a single strand in each helix is annealed to the complementary strand in the other helix. The Holliday junction is a tetrahedral junction structure that can be moved along the pair of chromosomes, swapping one strand for another. The recombination reaction is then halted by cleavage of the junction and re-ligation of the released DNA.

Evolution

DNA contains the genetic information that allows all modern living things to function, grow and reproduce. However, it is unclear how long in the 4-billion-year history of life DNA has performed this function, as it has been proposed that the earliest forms of life may have used RNA as their genetic material. RNA may have acted as the central part of early cell metabolism as it can both transmit genetic information and carry out catalysis as part of ribozymes. This ancient RNA world where nucleic acid would have been used for both catalysis and genetics may have influenced the evolution of the current genetic code based on four nucleotide bases. This would occur, since the number of different bases in such an organism is a trade-off between a small number of bases increasing replication accuracy and a large number of bases increasing the catalytic efficiency of ribozymes. However, there is no direct evidence of ancient genetic systems, as recovery of DNA from most fossils is impossible. This is because DNA will survive in the environment for less than one million years and slowly degrades into short fragments in solution. Claims for older DNA have been made, most notably a report of the isolation of a viable bacterium from a salt crystal 250 million years old, but these claims are controversial.

Uses in technology

Genetic Engineering

Genetic engineering, also called genetic modification, is the direct human manipulation of an organism's genetic material in a way that does not occur under natural conditions. It involves the use of recombinant DNA techniques, but does not include traditional animal and plant breeding or mutagenesis. Any organism that is generated using these techniques is considered to be a genetically modified organism.

The first organisms genetically engineered were bacteria in 1973 and then mice in 1974. Insulin producing bacteria were commercialized in 1982 and genetically modified food has been sold since 1994. Producing genetically modified organisms or tissues is a multi-step process. It first involves the isolating and copying the genetic material of interest; if necessary, changes to genetic sequence may be introduced. A construct may be built containing all the genetic elements for correct expression in a vector.

This vector construct is then introduced into the host organism in a process called transformation, transfection or transduction. Successfully transformed organisms or tissues are then selectively grown, usually by growing material in conditions which require the presence of a gene in the inserted material for survival. Genetic engineering techniques have been applied to various industries, with some success.

Medicines such as insulin and human growth hormone are now produced in bacteria, experimental mice such as the oncomouse and the knockout mouse are being used for research purposes and insect resistant and/or herbicide tolerant crops have been commercialized. Plants that contain drugs and vaccines, animals with beneficial proteins in their milk and stress tolerant crops are currently being developed.

Forensics

Forensic scientists can use DNA in blood, semen, skin, saliva or hair found at a crime scene to identify a matching DNA of an individual, such as a perpetrator. This process is formally termed DNA profiling, but may also be called "genetic fingerprinting". In DNA profiling, the lengths of variable sections of repetitive DNA, such as short tandem repeats and minisatellites, are compared between people.

This method is usually an extremely reliable technique for identifying a matching DNA.However, identification can be complicated if the scene is contaminated with DNA from several people.DNA profiling was developed in 1984 by British geneticist Sir Alec Jeffreys,and first used in forensic science to convict Colin Pitchfork in the 1988 Enderby murders case.

People convicted of certain types of crimes may be required to provide a sample of DNA for a database. This has helped investigators solve old cases where only a DNA sample was obtained from the scene. DNA profiling can also be used to identify victims of mass casualty incidents.On the other hand, many convicted people have been released from prison on the basis of DNA techniques, which were not available when a crime had originally been committed.

Bioinformatics

Bioinformatics involves the manipulation, searching, and data mining of biological data, and this includes DNA sequence data. The development of techniques to store and search DNA sequences have led to widely applied advances in computer science, especially string searching algorithms, machine learning and database theory.String searching or matching algorithms, which find an occurrence of a sequence of letters inside a larger sequence of letters, were developed to search for specific sequences of nucleotides. The DNA sequenced may be aligned with other DNA sequences to identify homologous sequences and locate the specific mutations that make them distinct.

These techniques, especially multiple sequence alignment, are used in studying phylogenetic relationships and protein function. Data sets representing entire genomes' worth of DNA sequences, such as those produced by the Human Genome Project, are difficult to use without the annotations that identify the locations of genes and regulatory elements on each chromosome. Regions of DNA sequence that have the characteristic patterns associated with protein- or RNA-coding genes can be identified by gene finding algorithms, which allow researchers to predict the presence of particular gene products and their possible functions in an organism even before they have been isolated experimentally.Entire genomes may also be compared which can shed light on the evolutionary history of particular organism and permit the examination of complex evolutionary events.

DNA Nanotechnology

DNA nanotechnology uses the unique molecular recognition properties of DNA and other nucleic acids to create self-assembling branched DNA complexes with useful properties.DNA is thus used as a structural material rather than as a carrier of biological information. This has led to the creation of two-dimensional periodic lattices (both tile-based as well as using the "DNA origami" method) as well as three-dimensional structures in the shapes of polyhedra. Nanomechanical devices and algorithmic self-assembly have also been demonstrated,and these DNA structures have been used to template the arrangement of other molecules such as gold nanoparticles and streptavidin proteins.

History and Anthropology

Because DNA collects mutations over time, which are then inherited, it contains historical information, and, by comparing DNA sequences, geneticists can infer the evolutionary history of organisms, their phylogeny. This field of phylogenetics is a powerful tool in evolutionary biology. If DNA sequences within a species are compared, population geneticists can learn the history of particular populations. This can be used in studies ranging from ecological genetics to anthropology; For example, DNA evidence is being used to try to identify the Ten Lost Tribes of Israel. DNA has also been used to look at modern family relationships, such as establishing family relationships between the descendants of Sally Hemings and Thomas Jefferson. This usage is closely related to the use of DNA in criminal investigations. Indeed, some criminal investigations have been solved when DNA from crime scenes has matched relatives of the guilty individual.

PROTEIN SYNTHESIS

During the 1950s and 1960s it became apparent that DNA is essential in the synthesis of proteins. Proteins are used as structural materials in the cells and function as enzymes. In addition, many specialized proteins function in cellular activities. For example, in bacteria, flagella and pili are composed of protein.

The genetic code

The key element of a protein molecule is how the amino acids are linked. The sequences of amino acids, determined by genetic codes in DNA, distinguish one protein from another. The genetic code consists of the sequence of nitrogenous bases in the DNA. How the nitrogenous base code is translated to an amino acid sequence in a protein is the basis for protein synthesis. In order for protein synthesis to occur, several essential materials must be present.

One is a supply of the 20 amino acids which make up most proteins. Another essential element is a series of enzymes that will function in the process. DNA and another form of nucleic acid called ribonucleic acid (RNA) are also essential. RNA carries instructions from the nuclear DNA into the cytoplasm, where protein is synthesized. RNA is similar to DNA, with three exceptions. First, the carbohydrate in RNA is ribose rather than deoxyribose. Second, RNA nucleotides contain the pyrimidine uracil rather than thymine. And third, RNA is usually single-stranded.

Types of RNA

In the synthesis of protein, three types of RNA are required. The first is called ribosomal RNA (rRNA) and is used to manufacture ribosomes. Ribosomes are ultramicroscopic particles of rRNA and protein where amino acids are linked to one another during the synthesis of proteins. Ribosomes may exist along the membranes of the endoplasmic reticulum in eukaryotic cells or free in the cytoplasm of prokaryotic cells.

A second important type of RNA is transfer RNA (tRNA), which is used to carry amino acids to the ribosomes for protein synthesis. Molecules of tRNA exist free in the cytoplasm of cells. When protein synthesis is taking place, enzymes link tRNA to amino acids in a highly specific manner.

The third form of RNA is messenger RNA (mRNA), which receives the genetic code from DNA and carries it into the cytoplasm where protein synthesis takes place. In this way, a genetic code in the DNA can be used to synthesize a protein at a distant location at the ribosome. The synthesis of mRNA, tRNA, and rRNA is accomplished by an enzyme called RNA polymerase.

Transcription

Transcription is one of the first processes in the overall process of protein synthesis. In transcription, a strand of mRNA is synthesized using the genetic code of DNA. RNA polymerase binds to an area of a DNA molecule in the double helix (the other strand remains unused). The enzyme moves along the DNA strand and selects complementary bases from available nucleotides and positions them in an mRNA molecule just as to the principle of complementary base pairing. The chain of mRNA lengthens until a stop code is received.

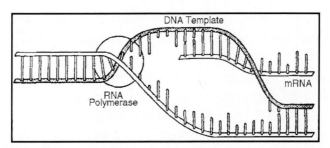

Fig. The Synthesis of mRNA using a Strand of DNA as a Template.

The nucleotides of the DNA strands are read in groups of three. Each triplet is called a codon. Thus, a codon may be CGA, or TTA, or GCT, or any other combination of the four bases, depending on their sequence in the DNA strand.

The mRNA molecule consists of a series of codons received from the genetic message in the DNA. Once the stop codon has been reached, the mRNA molecule leaves the DNA molecule, and the DNA molecule rewinds to form a double helix. Meanwhile, the mRNA molecule proceeds thorough the cellular cytoplasm towards the ribosomes.

Translation

Translation is the process in which the genetic code will be "translated" to an amino acid sequence in a protein. The process begins with the arrival of the mRNA molecule at the ribosomes. While mRNA was being synthesized, tRNA molecules were uniting with their specific amino acids just as to the activity of specific enzymes. The tRNA molecules then began transporting their amino acids to the ribosomes to meet the mRNA molecule.

After it arrives at the ribosomes, the mRNA molecule exposes its bases in sets of three, the codons. Each codon has a complementary codon called an anticodon on a tRNA molecule. When the codon of the mRNA molecule complements the anticodon on a tRNA molecule, the latter places the particular amino acid in that position. Then the next codon of the mRNA is exposed, and the complementary anticodon of a tRNA molecule matches with it.

The amino acid carried by the second tRNA molecule is thus positioned next to the first amino acid, and the two are linked. At this point, the tRNA molecules release their amino acids and return to the cytoplasm to link up with new molecules of amino acid. The ribosome then moves farther down the mRNA molecule and exposes another codon which attracts another tRNA molecule with its anticodon. Another amino acid is brought into position. In this way, amino acids continue to be added to the growing chain until the ribosome has moved down to the end of the mRNA molecule. The sequence of codons on the mRNA molecule thus determines the sequence of amino acids in the protein being constructed.

Once the protein has been completely synthesized, it is removed from the ribosome for further processing. For example, the protein may be stored in the Golgi body of a eukaryotic cell before release, or a bacterium may release it as a toxin. The mRNA molecule is broken up and the nucleotides are returned to the nucleus. The tRNA molecules return to the cytoplasm to unite with fresh molecules of amino acids, and the ribosome awaits the arrival of a new mRNA molecule.

Gene control

The process of protein synthesis does not occur constantly in the cell, but rather at intervals followed by periods of genetic "silence." Thus, the process of gene expression is regulated and controlled by the cell. The control of gene expression can occur at several levels in the cell. For example, genes rarely operate during mitosis. Other levels of gene control can occur at transcription, when certain segments of DNA increase and accelerate the activity of nearby genes.

After transcription has taken place, the mRNA molecule can be altered to regulate gene activity. For example, it has been found that eukaryotic mRNA contains many useless bits of RNA that are removed in the production of the final mRNA molecule. These useless bits of nucleic acid are called introns. The remaining pieces of mRNA, called exons, are then spliced to form the final mRNA molecule. Bacterial mRNA lacks introns.

The concept of gene control has been researched thoroughly in bacteria. In these microorganisms, genes have been identified as structural genes, regulator genes, and control regions. The three units form a functional unit called the operon. The operon has been examined in close detail in certain bacteria. It has been found that certain carbohydrates can induce the presence of the enzymes needed to digest those carbohydrates.

For example, when lactose is present, bacteria synthesize the enzymes needed to break it down. Lactose acts as an inducer molecule in the following way: In the absence of lactose, a regulator gene produces a repressor protein, which binds to a control region called the operator site. This binding prevents the structural genes from encoding the enzyme for lactose digestion. When lactose is present, however, it binds to the repressor protein and thereby removes the repressor at the operator site. With the operator site free, the structural genes are released to produce their lactose-digesting enzyme.

RECOMBINANT DNA AND BIOTECHNOLOGY

Biotechnology is an industrial process that uses the scientific research on DNA for practical benefits. Biotechnology is synonymous with genetic engineering because the genes of an organism are changed during the process and the DNA of the organism is recombined. Recombinant DNA and biotechnology can be used to form proteins not normally produced in a cell. In addition, bacteria that carry recombinant DNA can be released into the environment to increase the fertility of the soil, serve as an insecticide, or relieve pollution.

Tools of biotechnology

The basic process of recombinant DNA technology revolves around the activity of DNA in the synthesis of protein. By intervening in this process, scientists can change the nature of the DNA and of the gene make-up of an organism. By inserting genes into the genome of an organism, the scientist can induce the organism to produce a protein it does not normally produce.The technology of recombinant DNA has been made possible in part by extensive research on microorganisms during the last century.

One important microorganism in recombinant DNA research is Escherichia coli (E. coli). The biochemistry and genetics of E. coli are well known, and its DNA has been isolated and made to accept new genes. The DNA can then be forced into fresh cells of E. coli, and the bacteria will begin to produce the proteins specified by the foreign genes. Such altered bacteria are said to have been transformed.

Interest in recombinant DNA and biotechnology heightened considerably in the 1960s and 1970s with the discovery of restriction enzymes. These enzymes catalyze the opening of a DNA molecule at a "restricted" point, regardless of the DNA's source. Moreover, certain restriction enzymes leave dangling ends of DNA molecules at the point where the DNA is open. (The most commonly used restriction enzyme is named EcoRl.) Foreign DNA can then be combined with the carrier DNA at this point. An enzyme called DNA ligase is used to form a permanent link between the dangling ends of the DNA molecules at the point of union.

Pharmaceutical products

Gene defects in humans can lead to deficiencies in proteins such as insulin, human growth hormone, and Factor VIII. These protein deficiencies may lead to problems such as diabetes, dwarfism, and impaired blood clotting, respectively. Missing proteins can now be replaced by proteins manufactured through biotechnology. For insulin production, two protein chains are encoded by separate genes in plasmids inserted into bacteria. The protein chains are then chemically joined to form the final insulin product. Human growth hormone is also produced within bacteria, but special techniques are used because the bacteria do not usually produce human proteins. Therapeutic proteins produced by biotechnology include a clot-dissolving protein called tissue plasminogen activator (TPA) and interferon.

This antiviral protein is produced within *E. coli* cells. Interferon is currently used against certain types of cancers and for certain skin conditions. Vaccines represent another application of recombinant DNA technology. For instance, the hepatitis B vaccine now in use is composed of viral protein manufactured by yeast cells, which have been recombined with viral genes. The vaccine is safe because it contains no viral particles. Experimental vaccines against AIDS are being produced in the same way.

Diagnostic testing

Recombinant DNA and biotechnology have opened a new era of diagnostic testing and have made detecting many genetic diseases possible. The basic tool of DNA analyses is a fragment of DNA called the DNA probe. A DNA probe is a relatively small, single-stranded fragment of DNA that recognizes and binds to a complementary section of DNA in a complex mixture of DNA molecules. The probe mingles with the mixture of DNA and unites with the target DNA much like a left hand unites with the right. Once the probe unites with its target, it emits a signal such as radioactivity to indicate that a reaction has occurred. To work effectively, a sufficiently large amount of target DNA must be available. To increase the amount of available DNA, a process called the polymerase chain reaction (PCR) is used.

In a highly automated machine, the target DNA is combined with enzymes, nucleotides, and a primer DNA. In geometric fashion, the enzymes synthesize copies of the target DNA, so that in a few hours billions of molecules of DNA exist where only a few were before. Using DNA probes and PCR, scientists are now able to detect the DNA associated with HIV (and AIDS), Lyme disease, and genetic diseases such as cystic fibrosis, muscular dystrophy, Huntington's disease, and fragile X syndrome.

Gene therapy

Gene therapy is a recombinant DNA process in which cells are taken from the patient, altered by adding genes, and replaced in the patient, where the genes provide the genetic codes for proteins the patient is lacking. In the early 1990s, gene therapy was used to correct a deficiency of the enzyme adenosine deaminase (ADA).

Blood cells called lymphocytes were removed from the bone marrow of two children; then genes for ADA production were inserted into the cells using viruses as vectors. Finally, the cells were reinfused to the bodies of the two children. Once established in the bodies, the gene-altered cells began synthesizing the enzyme ADA and alleviated the deficiency. Gene therapy has also been performed with patients with melanoma (a virulent skin cancer). In this case, lymphocytes that normally attack tumors are isolated in the patients and treated with genes for an anticancer protein called tumor necrosis factor. The genealtered lymphocytes are then reinfused to the patients, where they produce the new protein which helps destroy cancer cells. Approximately 2000 single-gene defects are believed to exist, and patients with these defects may be candidates for gene therapy.

DNA fingerprinting

The use of DNA probes and the development of retrieval techniques have made it possible to match DNA molecules to one another for identification purposes. This process has been used in a forensic procedure called DNA fingerprinting. The use of DNA fingerprinting depends upon the presence of repeating base sequences that exist in the human genome.

The repeating sequences are called restriction fragment length polymorphisms (RFLPs). As the pattern of RFLPs is unique for every individual, it can be used as a molecular fingerprint. To perform DNA fingerprinting, DNA is obtained from an individual's blood cells, hair fibres, skin fragments, or other tissue. The DNA is extracted from the cells and digested with enzymes. The resulting fragments are separated by a process called electrophoresis. These separated DNA fragments are tested for characteristic RFLPs using DNA probes. A statistical evaluation enables the forensic pathologist to compare a suspect's DNA with the DNA recovered at a crime scene and to assert with a degree of certainty (usually 99 per cent) that the suspect was at the crime scene.

DNA and agriculture

Although plants are more difficult to work with than bacteria, gene insertions can be made into single plant cells, and the cells can then be cultivated to form a mature plant. The major method for inserting genes is through the plasmids of a bacterium called Agrobacterium tumefaciens. This bacterium invades plant cells, and its plasmids insert into plant chromosomes carrying the genes for tumor induction.

Scientists remove the tumor-inducing genes and obtain a plasmid that unites with the plant cell without causing any harm. Recombinant DNA and biotechnology have been used to increase the efficiency of plant growth by increasing the efficiency of the plant's ability to fix nitrogen. Scientists have obtained the genes for nitrogen fixation from bacteria and have incorporated those genes into plant cells.

By obtaining nitrogen directly from the atmosphere, the plants can synthesize their own proteins without intervention of bacteria as normally needed. DNA technology has also been used to increase plant resistance to disease. The genes for an insecticide have been obtained from the bacterium Bacillus thuringiensis and inserted into plants to allow them to resist caterpillars and other pests. In addition, plants have been reengineered to produce the capsid protein that encloses viruses. These proteins lend resistance to the plants against viral disease.

The human genome

One of the most ambitious scientific endeavors of the twentieth century was the effort to sequence the nitrogenous bases in the human genome. Begun in 1990 and completed in 2003, the effort encompassed 13 years of work at a cost of approximately $3 billion. Knowing the content of the human genome is helping researchers devise new diagnostics and treatments for genetic diseases and will also be of value to developmental biologists, evolutionary biologists, and comparative biologists. In addition to learning the genome of humans, the project has also studied numerous bacteria. By 1995, the genomes of two bacteria had been completely deciphered (Haemophilus influenzae and Mycoplasma genitalium), and by 1996, the genome of the yeast Saccharomyces cerevisiae was known. The Human Genome Project is one of colossal magnitude that will have an impact on many branches of science for decades to come. The project remains the crowning achievement of DNA research in the twentieth century and the bedrock for research in the twenty-first.

MICROORGANISM

A microorganism or microbe is an organism that is unicellular or lives in a colony of cellular organisms. The study of microorganisms is called microbiology, a subject that began with Anton van Leeuwenhoek's discovery of microorganisms in 1675, using a microscope of his own design. Microorganisms are very diverse; they include bacteria, fungi, archaea, and protists; microscopic plants; and animals such as plankton and the planarian. Some microbiologists also include viruses, but others consider these as non-living.

Most microorganisms are unicellular but this is not universal, since some multicellular organisms are microscopic, while some unicellular protists and bacteria, like Thiomargarita namibiensis, are macroscopic and visible to the naked eye. Microorganisms live in all parts of the biosphere where there is liquid water, including soil, hot springs, on the ocean floor, high in the atmosphere and deep inside rocks within the Earth's crust.

Microorganisms are critical to nutrient recycling in ecosystems as they act as decomposers. As some microorganisms can fix nitrogen, they are a vital part of the nitrogen cycle, and recent studies indicate that airborne microbes may play a role in precipitation and weather. Microbes are also exploited by people in biotechnology, both in traditional food and beverage preparation, and in modern technologies based on genetic engineering. However, pathogenic microbes are harmful, since they invade and grow within other organisms, causing diseases that kill people, other animals and plants.

History

Evolution

Single-celled microorganisms were the first forms of life to develop on Earth, approximately 3–4 billion years ago. Further evolution was slow, and for about 3 billion years in the Precambrian eon, all organisms were microscopic. So, for most of the history of life on Earth the only forms of life were microorganisms. Bacteria, algae and fungi have been identified in amber that is 220 million years old, which shows that the morphology of microorganisms has changed little since the Triassic period.

Most microorganisms can reproduce rapidly and microbes such as bacteria can also freely exchange genes by conjugation, transformation and transduction between widely-divergent species. This horizontal gene transfer, coupled with a high mutation rate and many other means of genetic variation, allows microorganisms to swiftly evolve to survive in new environments and respond to environmental stresses. This rapid evolution is important in medicine, as it has led to the recent development of 'super-bugs' — pathogenic bacteria that are resistant to modern antibiotics.

Pre-microbiology

The possibility that microorganisms exist was discussed for many centuries before their actual discovery in the 17th century. The existence of unseen microbiological life was postulated by Jainism which is based on Mahavira's teachings as early as 6th century BCE. Paul Dundas notes that Mahavira asserted existence of unseen microbiological creatures living in earth, water, air and fire. Jain scriptures also describe nigodas which are sub-microscopic creatures living in large clusters and having a very short life and are said to pervade each and every part of universe, even in tissues of plants and flesh of animals. However, the earliest known idea to indicate the possibility of diseases spreading by yet unseen organisms was that of the Roman scholar Marcus Terentius Varro in a 1st century BC book titled On Agriculture in which he warns against locating a homestead near swamps:

- …and because there are bred certain minute creatures which cannot be seen by the eyes, which float in the air and enter the body through the mouth and nose and there cause serious diseases.

In The Canon of Medicine, Avicenna stated that bodily secretion is contaminated by foul foreign earthly bodies before being infected. He also hypothesized that tuberculosis and other diseases might be contagious, *i.e.* that they were infectious diseases, and used quarantine to limit their spread. When the Black Death bubonic plague reached Andalusia in Spain, in the 14th century, Ibn Khatima wrote that infectious diseases were caused by contagious "minute bodies" that enter the human body. Later, in 1546, Girolamo Fracastoro proposed that epidemic diseases were caused by transferable seedlike entities that could transmit infection by direct or indirect contact, or even without contact over long distances. All these early claims about the existence of microorganisms were speculative and were not based on any data or science. Microorganisms were neither proven, observed, nor correctly and accurately described until the 17th century. The reason for this was that all these early studies lacked the microscope.

History of Microorganisms' Discovery

Anton van Leeuwenhoek was one of the first people to observe microorganisms, using a microscope of his own design, and made one of the most important contributions to biology. Robert Hooke was the first to use a microscope to observe living things; his 1665 book Micrographia contained descriptions of plant cells. Before Leeuwenhoek's discovery of microorganisms in 1675, it had been a mystery why grapes could be turned into wine, milk into cheese, or why food would spoil. Leeuwenhoek did not make the connection between these processes and microorganisms, but using a microscope, he did establish that there were forms of life that were not visible to the naked eye. Leeuwenhoek's discovery, along with subsequent observations by Lazzaro Spallanzani and Louis Pasteur, ended the long-held belief that life spontaneously appeared from non-living substances during the process of spoilage.

Lazzaro Spallanzani found that boiling broth would sterilise it and kill any microorganisms in it. He also found that new microorganisms could only settle in a broth if the broth was exposed to the air. Louis Pasteur expanded upon Spallanzani's findings by exposing boiled broths to the air, in vessels that contained a filter to prevent all particles from passing through to the growth medium, and also in vessels with no filter at all, with air being admitted via a curved tube that would not allow dust particles to come in contact with the broth. By boiling the broth beforehand, Pasteur ensured that no microorganisms survived within the broths at the beginning of his experiment. Nothing grew in the broths in the course of Pasteur's experiment. This meant that the living organisms that grew in such broths came from outside, as spores on dust, rather than spontaneously generated within the broth. Thus, Pasteur dealt the death blow to the theory of spontaneous generation and supported germ theory.

In 1876, Robert Koch established that microbes can cause disease. He found that the blood of cattle who were infected with anthrax always had large numbers of Bacillus anthracis. Koch found that he could transmit anthrax from one animal to another by taking a small sample of blood from the infected animal and injecting it into a healthy one, and this caused the healthy animal to become sick. He also found that he could grow the bacteria in a nutrient broth, then inject it into a healthy animal, and cause illness.

Based on these experiments, he devised criteria for establishing a causal link between a microbe and a disease and these are now known as Koch's postulates. Although these postulates cannot be applied in all cases, they do retain historical importance to the development of scientific thought and are still being used today.

CLASSIFICATION AND STRUCTURE

Microorganisms can be found almost anywhere in the taxonomic organization of life on the planet. Bacteria and archaea are almost always microscopic, while a number of eukaryotes are also microscopic, including most protists, some fungi, as well as some animals and plants. Viruses are generally regarded as not living and therefore are not microbes, although the field of microbiology also encompasses the study of viruses.

Prokaryotes

Prokaryotes are organisms that lack a cell nucleus and the other membrane bound organelles. They are almost always unicellular, although some species such as myxobacteria can aggregate into complex structures as part of their life cycle.Consisting of two domains, bacteria and archaea, the prokaryotes are the most diverse and abundant group of organisms on Earth and inhabit practically all environments where some liquid water is available and the temperature is below +140 °C. They are found in sea water, soil, air, animals' gastrointestinal tracts, hot springs and even deep beneath the Earth's crust in rocks. Practically all surfaces which have not been specially sterilized are covered by prokaryotes. The number of prokaryotes on Earth is estimated to be around five million trillion trillion, or 5×10, accounting for at least half the biomass on Earth.

Bacteria

Bacteria are practically all invisible to the naked eye, with a few extremely rare exceptions, such as Thiomargarita namibiensis. They lack membrane-bound organelles, and can function and reproduce as individual cells, but often aggregate in multicellular colonies. Their genome is usually a single loop of DNA, although they can also harbor small pieces of DNA called plasmids. These plasmids can be transferred between cells through bacterial conjugation. Bacteria are surrounded by a cell wall, which provides strength and rigidity to their cells. They reproduce by binary fission or sometimes by budding, but do not undergo sexual reproduction. Some species form extraordinarily resilient spores, but for bacteria this is a mechanism for survival, not reproduction. Under optimal conditions bacteria can grow extremely rapidly and can double as quickly as every 10 minutes.

Archaea

Archaea are also single-celled organisms that lack nuclei. In the past, the differences between bacteria and archaea were not recognised and archaea were classified with bacteria as part of the kingdom Monera. However, in 1990 the microbiologist Carl Woese proposed the three-domain system that divided living things into bacteria, archaea and eukaryotes. Archaea differ from bacteria in both their genetics and biochemistry. For example, while bacterial cell membranes are made from phosphoglycerides with ester bonds, archaean membranes are made of ether lipids. Archaea were originally described in extreme environments, such as hot springs, but have since been found in all types of habitats. Only now are scientists beginning to realise how common archaea are in the environment, with crenarchaeota being the most common form of life in the ocean, dominating ecosystems below 150 m in depth. These organisms are also common in soil and play a vital role in ammonia oxidation.

Eukaryotes

Most living things which are visible to the naked eye in their adult form are eukaryotes, including humans. However, a large number of eukaryotes are also microorganisms. Unlike bacteria and archaea, eukaryotes contain organelles such as the cell nucleus, the Golgi apparatus and mitochondria in their cells. The nucleus is an organelle which houses the DNA that makes up a cell's genome. DNA itself is arranged in complex chromosomes. Mitochondria are organelles vital in metabolism as they are the site of the citric acid cycle and oxidative phosphorylation. They evolved from symbiotic bacteria and retain a remnant genome. Like bacteria, plant cells have cell walls, and contain organelles such as chloroplasts in addition to the organelles in other eukaryotes. Chloroplasts produce energy from light by photosynthesis, and were also originally symbiotic bacteria. Unicellular eukaryotes are those eukaryotic organisms that consist of a single cell throughout their life cycle. This qualification is significant since most multicellular eukaryotes consist of a single cell called a zygote at the beginning of their life cycles. Microbial eukaryotes can be either haploid or diploid, and some organisms have multiple cell nuclei. However, not all microorganisms are unicellular as some microscopic eukaryotes are made from multiple cells. Of eukaryotic groups, the protists are most commonly unicellular and microscopic. This is a highly diverse group of organisms that are not easy to classify. Several algae species are multicellular protists, and slime molds have unique life cycles that involve switching between unicellular, colonial, and multicellular forms. The number of species of protozoa is uncertain, since we may have identified only a small proportion of the diversity in this group of organisms.

Animals

Mostly animals are multicellular, but some are too small to be seen by the naked eye. Microscopic arthropods include dust mites and spider mites. Microscopic crustaceans include copepods and the cladocera, while many nematodes are too small to be seen with the naked eye. Another particularly common group of microscopic animals are the rotifers, which are filter feeders that are usually found in fresh water. Micro-animals reproduce both sexually and asexually and may reach new habitats as eggs that survive harsh environments that would kill the adult animal. However, some simple animals, such as rotifers and nematodes, can dry out completely and remain dormant for long periods of time.

Fungi

The fungi have several unicellular species, such as baker's yeast and fission yeast. Some fungi, such as the pathogenic yeast Candida albicans, can undergo phenotypic switching and grow as single cells in some environments, and filamentous hyphae in others. Fungi reproduce both asexually, by budding or binary fission, as well by producing spores, which are called conidia when produced asexually, or basidiospores when produced sexually.

Plants

The green algae are a large group of photosynthetic eukaryotes that include many microscopic organisms. Although some green algae are classified as protists, others such as charophyta are classified with embryophyte plants, which are the most familiar group of land plants. Algae can grow as single cells, or in long chains of cells. The green algae include unicellular and colonial flagellates, usually but not always with two flagella per cell, as well as various colonial, coccoid, and filamentous forms. In the Charales, which are the algae most closely related to higher plants, cells differentiate into several distinct tissues within the organism. There are about 6000 species of green algae.

Habitats and ecology

Microorganisms are found in almost every habitat present in nature. Even in hostile environments such as the poles, deserts, geysers, rocks, and the deep sea. Some types of microorganisms have adapted to the extreme conditions and sustained colonies; these organisms are known as extremophiles. Extremophiles have been isolated from rocks as much as 7 kilometres below the Earth's surface, and it has been suggested that the amount of living organisms below the Earth's surface may be comparable with the amount of life on or above the surface. Extremophiles have been known to survive for a prolonged time in a vacuum, and can be highly resistant to radiation, which may even allow them to survive in space.

Many types of microorganisms have intimate symbiotic relationships with other larger organisms; some of which are mutually beneficial while others can be damaging to the host organism. If microorganisms can cause disease in a host they are known as pathogens.

Extremophiles

Extremophiles are microorganisms which have adapted so that they can survive and even thrive in conditions that are normally fatal to most life-forms.

For example, some species have been found in the following extreme environments:

- *Temperature*: As high as 130 °C, as low as –17 °C
- *Acidity/alkalinity*: Less than pH 0, up to pH 11.5
- *Salinity*: Up to saturation
- *Pressure*: Up to 1,000-2,000 atm, down to 0 atm
- *Radiation*: Up to 5kGy

Extremophiles are significant in different ways. They extend terrestrial life into much of the Earth's hydrosphere, crust and atmosphere, their specific evolutionary adaptation mechanisms to their extreme environment can be exploited in bio-technology, and their very existence under such extreme conditions increases the potential for extraterrestrial life.

Soil Microbes

The nitrogen cycle in soils depends on the fixation of atmospheric nitrogen. One way this can occur is in the nodules in the roots of legumes that contain symbiotic bacteria of the genera Rhizobium, Mesorhizobium, Sinorhizobium, Bradyrhizobium, and Azorhizobium.

Symbiotic Microbes

Symbiotic microbes such as fungi and algae form an association in lichen.

Certain fungi form mycorrhizal symbioses with trees that increase the supply of nutrients to the tree.

Importance

Microorganisms are vital to humans and the environment, as they participate in the Earth's element cycles such as the carbon cycle and nitrogen cycle, as well as fulfilling other vital roles in virtually all ecosystems, such as recycling other organisms' dead remains and waste products through decomposition. Microbes also have an important place in most higher-order multicellular organisms as symbionts. Many blame the failure of Biosphere 2 on an improper balance of microbes.

- *Use in food*: Microorganisms are used in brewing, winemaking, baking, pickling and other food-making processes. They are also used to control the fermentation process in the production of cultured dairy products such as yogurt and cheese. The cultures also provide flavour and aroma, and inhibit undesirable organisms.

- *Use in water treatment*: Specially-cultured microbes are used in the biological treatment of sewage and industrial waste effluent, a process known as bioaugmentation.

- *Use in energy*: Microbes are used in fermentation to produce ethanol, and in biogas reactors to produce methane. Scientists are researching the use of algae to produce liquid fuels, and bacteria to convert various forms of agricultural and urban waste into usable fuels.

- *Use in science*: Microbes are also essential tools in biotechnology, biochemistry, genetics, and molecular biology. The yeasts and fission yeast are important model organisms in science, since they are simple eukaryotes that can be grown rapidly in large numbers and are easily manipulated. They are particularly valuable in genetics, genomics and proteomics. Microbes can be harnessed for uses such as creating steroids and treating skin diseases. Scientists are also considering using microbes for living fuel cells, and as a solution for pollution.

- *Use in warfare*: In the Middle Ages, diseased corpses were thrown into castles during sieges using catapults or other siege engines. Individuals near the corpses were exposed to the deadly pathogen and were likely to spread that pathogen to others.

IMPORTANCE IN HUMAN HEALTH

- *Human digestion*: Microorganisms can form an endosymbiotic relationship with other, larger organisms. For example, the bacteria that live within the human digestive system contribute to gut immunity, synthesise vitamins such as folic acid and biotin, and ferment complex indigestible carbohydrates.

• *Diseases and immunology*: Microorganisms are the cause of many infectious diseases. The organisms involved include pathogenic bacteria, causing diseases such as plague, tuberculosis and anthrax; protozoa, causing diseases such as malaria, sleeping sickness and toxoplasmosis; and also fungi causing diseases such as ringworm, candidiasis or histoplasmosis. However, other diseases such as influenza, yellow fever or AIDS are caused by pathogenic viruses, which are not usually classified as living organisms and are not therefore microorganisms by the strict definition. As of 2007, no clear examples of archaean pathogens are known, although a relationship has been proposed between the presence of some methanogens and human periodontal disease.

THE BACTERIAL CHROMOSOME AND PLASMID

While eukaryotes have two or more chromosomes, prokaryotes such as bacteria possess a single chromosome composed of double-stranded DNA in a loop. The DNA is located in the nucleoid of the cell and is not associated with protein. In *Escherichia coli*, the length of the chromosome, when open, is many times the length of the cell. Many bacteria (and some yeasts or other fungi) also possess looped bits of DNA known as plasmids, which exist and replicate independently of the chromosome. Plasmids have relatively few genes (fewer than 30). The genetic information of the plasmid is usually not essential to survival of the host bacteria. Plasmids can be removed from the host cell in the process of curing. Curing may occur spontaneously or may be induced by treatments such as ultraviolet light. Certain plasmids, called episomes, may be integrated into the bacterial chromosome. Others contain genes for certain types of pili and are able to transfer copies of themselves to other bacteria. Such plasmids are referred to as conjugative plasmids.

A special plasmid called a fertility (F) factor plays an important role in conjugation. The F factor contains genes that encourage cellular attachment during conjugation and accelerate plasmid transfer between conjugating bacterial cells. Those cells contributing DNA are called F^+ (donor) cells, while those receiving DNA are the F^- (recipient) cells. The F factor can exist outside the bacterial chromosome or may be integrated into the chromosome.

Plasmids contain genes that impart antibiotic resistance. Up to eight genes for resisting eight different antibiotics may be found on a single plasmid. Genes that encode a series of bacteriocins are also found on plasmids. Bacteriocins are bacterial proteins capable of destroying other bacteria. Still other plasmids increase the pathogenicity of their host bacteria because the plasmid contains genes for toxin synthesis. Transposable elements.

Transposable elements, also known as transposons, are segments of DNA that move about within the chromosome and establish new genetic sequences. First discovered by Barbara McClintock in the 1940s, transposons behave somewhat like lysogenic viruses except that they cannot exist apart from the chromosome or reproduce themselves.

The simplest transposons, insertion sequences, are short sequences of DNA bounded at both ends by identical sequences of nucleotides in reverse orientation (inverted repeats). Insertion sequences can insert within a gene and cause a rearrangement mutation of the genetic material. If the sequence carries a stop codon, it may block transcription of the DNA during protein synthesis. Insertion sequences may also encourage the movement of drug-resistance genes between plasmids and chromosomes.

MUTATION

In molecular biology and genetics, mutations are changes in a genomic sequence: the DNA sequence of a cell's genome or the DNA or RNA sequence of a virus. Mutations are caused by radiation, viruses, transposons and mutagenic chemicals, as well as errors that occur during meiosis or DNA replication. They can also be induced by the organism itself, by cellular processes such as hypermutation. Mutation can result in several different types of change in DNA sequences; these can either have no effect, alter the product of a gene, or prevent the gene from functioning properly or completely. Studies in the fly Drosophila melanogaster suggest that if a mutation changes a protein produced by a gene, this will probably be harmful, with about 70 per cent of these mutations having damaging effects, and the remainder being either neutral or weakly beneficial.

Due to the damaging effects that mutations can have on genes, organisms have mechanisms such as DNA repair to remove mutations. Therefore, the optimal mutation rate for a species is a trade-off between costs of a high mutation rate, such as deleterious mutations, and the metabolic costs of maintaining systems to reduce the mutation rate, such as DNA repair enzymes. Viruses that use RNA as their genetic material have rapid mutation rates, which can be an advantage since these viruses will evolve constantly and rapidly, and thus evade the defensive responses of *e.g.* the human immune system.

Description

Mutations can involve large sections of DNA becoming duplicated, usually through genetic recombination. These duplications are a major source of raw material for evolving new genes, with tens to hundreds of genes duplicated in animal genomes every million years. Most genes belong to larger families of genes of shared ancestry. Novel genes are produced by several methods, commonly through the duplication and mutation of an ancestral gene, or by recombining parts of different genes to form new combinations with new functions. Here, domains act as modules, each with a particular and independent function, that can be mixed together to produce genes encoding new proteins with novel properties. For example, the human eye uses four genes to make structures that sense light: three for color vision and one for night vision; all four arose from a single ancestral gene.

Another advantage of duplicating a gene (or even an entire genome) is that this increases redundancy; this allows one gene in the pair to acquire a new function while the other copy performs the original function. Other types of mutation occasionally create new genes from previously noncoding DNA. Changes in chromosome number may involve even larger mutations, where segments of the DNA within chromosomes break and then rearrange.

For example, two chromosomes in the Homo genus fused to produce human chromosome 2; this fusion did not occur in the lineage of the other apes, and they retain these separate chromosomes. In evolution, the most important role of such chromosomal rearrangements may be to accelerate the divergence of a population into new species by making populations less likely to interbreed, and thereby preserving genetic differences between these populations.

Sequences of DNA that can move about the genome, such as transposons, make up a major fraction of the genetic material of plants and animals, and may have been important in the evolution of genomes. For example, more than a million copies of the Alu sequence are present in the human genome, and these sequences have now been recruited to perform functions such as regulating gene expression.

Another effect of these mobile DNA sequences is that when they move within a genome, they can mutate or delete existing genes and thereby produce genetic diversity. In multicellular organisms with dedicated reproductive cells, mutations can be subdivided into germ line mutations, which can be passed on to descendants through their reproductive cells, and somatic mutations (also called acquired mutations), which involve cells outside the dedicated reproductive group and which are not usually transmitted to descendants. If the organism can reproduce asexually through mechanisms such as cuttings or budding the distinction can become blurred. For example, plants can sometimes transmit somatic mutations to their descendants asexually or sexually where flower buds develop in somatically mutated parts of plants. A new mutation that was not inherited from either parent is called a de novo mutation.

The source of the mutation is unrelated to the consequence, although the consequences are related to which cells were mutated. Nonlethal mutations accumulate within the gene pool and increase the amount of genetic variation. The abundance of some genetic changes within the gene pool can be reduced by natural selection, while other "more favourable" mutations may accumulate and result in adaptive changes. For example, a butterfly may produce offspring with new mutations. The majority of these mutations will have no effect; but one might change the color of one of the butterfly's offspring, making it harder (or easier) for predators to see. If this color change is advantageous, the chance of this butterfly surviving and producing its own offspring are a little better, and over time the number of butterflies with this mutation may form a larger percentage of the population. Neutral mutations are defined as mutations whose effects do not influence the fitness of an individual. These can accumulate over time due to genetic drift. It is believed that the overwhelming majority of mutations have no significant effect on an organism's fitness. Also, DNA repair mechanisms are able to mend most changes before they become permanent mutations, and many organisms have mechanisms for eliminating otherwise permanently mutated somatic cells. Mutation is generally accepted by biologists as the mechanism by which natural selection acts, generating advantageous new traits that survive and multiply in offspring as well as disadvantageous traits, in less fit offspring, that tend to die out.

Causes

Two classes of mutations are spontaneous mutations (molecular decay) and induced mutations caused by mutagens.

Spontaneous mutations on the molecular level can be caused by:

- *Tautomerism*: A base is changed by the repositioning of a hydrogen atom, altering the hydrogen bonding pattern of that base resulting in incorrect base pairing during replication.

- *Depurination*: Loss of a purine base (A or G) to form an apurinic site (AP site).

- *Deamination*: Hydrolysis changes a normal base to an atypical base containing a keto group in place of the original amine group. Examples include C → U and A → HX (hypoxanthine), which can be corrected by DNA repair mechanisms; and 5MeC (5-methylcytosine) → T, which is less likely to be detected as a mutation because thymine is a normal DNA base.

- *Slipped strand mispairing*: Denaturation of the new strand from the template during replication, followed by renaturation in a different spot ("slipping"). This can lead to insertions or deletions.

Induced mutations on the molecular level can be caused by:

- Chemicals

  - Hydroxylamine NH_2OH

  - Base analogs (*e.g.* BrdU)

  - Alkylating agents (*e.g.* N-ethyl-N-nitrosourea) These agents can mutate both replicating and non-replicating DNA. In contrast, a base analog can only mutate the DNA when the analog is incorporated in replicating the DNA. Each of these classes of chemical mutagens has certain effects that then lead to transitions, transversions, or deletions.

  - Agents that form DNA adducts (*e.g.* ochratoxin A metabolites)

  - DNA intercalating agents (*e.g.* ethidium bromide)

  - DNA crosslinkers

  - Oxidative damage

  - Nitrous acid converts amine groups on A and C to diazo groups, altering their hydrogen bonding patterns which leads to incorrect base pairing during replication.

- Radiation

  - Ultraviolet radiation (nonionizing radiation). Two nucleotide bases in DNA–cytosine and thymine–are most vulnerable to radiation that can change their properties. UV light can induce adjacent pyrimidine bases in a DNA strand to become covalently joined as a pyrimidine dimer. UV radiation, particularly longer-wave UVA, can also cause oxidative damage to DNA.

  - Ionizing radiation

- Viral infections

DNA has so-called hotspots, where mutations occur up to 100 times more frequently than the normal mutation rate. A hotspot can be at an unusual base, *e.g.*, 5-methylcytosine. Mutation rates also vary across species. Evolutionary biologists have theorized that higher mutation rates are beneficial in some situations, because they allow organisms to evolve and therefore adapt more quickly to their environments. For example, repeated exposure of bacteria to antibiotics, and selection of resistant mutants, can result in the selection of bacteria that have a much higher mutation rate than the original population (mutator strains).

Classification of mutation types

By Effect on Structure

The sequence of a gene can be altered in a number of ways. Gene mutations have varying effects on health depending on where they occur and whether they alter the function of essential proteins.

Mutations in the structure of genes can be classified as:

- *Small-scale mutations, such as those affecting a small gene in one or a few nucleotides, including*:
  - Point mutations, often caused by chemicals or malfunction of DNA replication, exchange a single nucleotide for another. These changes are classified as transitions or transversions. Most common is the transition that exchanges a purine for a purine (A ↔ G) or a pyrimidine for a pyrimidine, (C ↔ T). A transition can be caused by nitrous acid, base mis-pairing, or mutagenic base analogs such as 5-bromo-2-deoxyuridine (BrdU). Less common is a transversion, which exchanges a purine for a pyrimidine or a pyrimidine for a purine (C/T ↔ A/G). An example of a transversion is adenine (A) being converted into a cytosine (C). A point mutation can be reversed by another point mutation, in which the nucleotide is changed back to its original state (true reversion) or by second-site reversion (a complementary mutation elsewhere that results in regained gene functionality). Point mutations that occur within the protein coding region of a gene may be classified into three kinds, depending upon what the erroneous codon codes for:
  1. *Silent mutations*: Which code for the same amino acid.
  2. *Missense mutations*: Which code for a different amino acid.

3. *Nonsense mutations*: Which code for a stop and can truncate the protein.

- Insertions add one or more extra nucleotides into the DNA. They are usually caused by transposable elements, or errors during replication of repeating elements (*e.g.* AT repeats). Insertions in the coding region of a gene may alter splicing of the mRNA (splice site mutation), or cause a shift in the reading frame (frameshift), both of which can significantly alter the gene product. Insertions can be reverted by excision of the transposable element.

- Deletions remove one or more nucleotides from the DNA. Like insertions, these mutations can alter the reading frame of the gene. They are generally irreversible: though exactly the same sequence might theoretically be restored by an insertion, transposable elements able to revert a very short deletion (say 1-2 bases) in any location are either highly unlikely to exist or do not exist at all. Note that a deletion is not the exact opposite of an insertion: the former is quite random while the latter consists of a specific sequence inserting at locations that are not entirely random or even quite narrowly defined.

• *Large-scale mutations in chromosomal structure, including*:
  - Amplifications (or gene duplications) leading to multiple copies of all chromosomal regions, increasing the dosage of the genes located within them.
  - Deletions of large chromosomal regions, leading to loss of the genes within those regions.
  - Mutations whose effect is to juxtapose previously separate pieces of DNA, potentially bringing together separate genes to form functionally distinct fusion genes (*e.g.* bcr-abl).

These include:

1. *Chromosomal translocations*: Interchange of genetic parts from nonhomologous chromo-somes.

2. *Interstitial deletions*: An intra-chromosomal deletion that removes a segment of DNA from a single chromosome, thereby apposing previously distant genes. For example, cells isolated from a human astrocytoma, a type of brain tumor, were found to have a chromosomal deletion removing sequences between the "fused in glioblastoma" gene and the receptor tyrosine kinase "ros", producing a fusion protein (FIG-ROS). The abnormal FIG-ROS

fusion protein has constitutively active kinase activity that causes oncogenic transformation (a transfor-mation from normal cells to cancer cells).

3. *Chromosomal inversions*: Reversing the orientation of a chromosomal segment.

- *Loss of heterozygosity*: Loss of one allele, either by a deletion or recombination event, in an organism that previously had two different alleles.

By Effect on Function

- Loss-of-function mutations are the result of gene product having less or no function. When the allele has a complete loss of function (null allele) it is often called an amorphic mutation. Phenotypes associated with such mutations are most often recessive. Exceptions are when the organism is haploid, or when the reduced dosage of a normal gene product is not enough for a normal phenotype (this is called haploinsufficiency).

- Gain-of-function mutations change the gene product such that it gains a new and abnormal function. These mutations usually have dominant phenotypes. Often called a neomorphic mutation.

- Dominant negative mutations (also called antimorphic mutations) have an altered gene product that acts antagonistically to the wild-type allele. These mutations usually result in an altered molecular function (often inactive) and are characterised by a dominant or semi-dominant phenotype.

- In humans, Marfan syndrome is an example of a dominant negative mutation occurring in an autosomal dominant disease.

In this condition, the defective glycoprotein product of the fibrillin gene (FBN1) antagonizes the product of the normal allele.

- Lethal mutations are mutations that lead to the death of the organisms which carry the mutations.

- A back mutation or reversion is a point mutation that restores the original sequence and hence the original phenotype.

By Effect on Fitness

In applied genetics it is usual to speak of mutations as either harmful or beneficial.

- A harmful mutation is a mutation that decreases the fitness of the organism.

- A beneficial mutation is a mutation that increases fitness of the organism, or which promotes traits that are desirable.

In theoretical population genetics, it is more usual to speak of such mutations as deleterious or advantageous.

In the neutral theory of molecular evolution, genetic drift is the basis for most variation at the molecular level.

- A neutral mutation has no harmful or beneficial effect on the organism. Such mutations occur at a steady rate, forming the basis for the molecular clock.

- A deleterious mutation has a negative effect on the phenotype, and thus decreases the fitness of the organism.

- An advantageous mutation has a positive effect on the phenotype, and thus increases the fitness of the organism.

- A nearly neutral mutation is a mutation that may be slightly deleterious or advantageous, although most nearly neutral mutations are slightly deleterious.

In reality, viewing the fitness effects of mutations in these discrete categories is an oversimplification. Attempts have been made to infer the distribution of fitness effects using mutagenesis experiments or theoretical models applied to molecular sequence data. However, the current distribution is still uncertain, and some aspects of the distribution likely vary between species.

By inheritance:

- Inheritable generic in pro-generic tissue or cells on path to be changed to gametes.

- Non inheritable somatic (*e.g.,* carcinogenic mutation)

- Non inheritable post mortem aDNA mutation in decaying remains.

By pattern of inheritance The human genome contains two copies of each gene– a paternal and a maternal allele:

- A heterozygous mutation is a mutation of only one allele.

- A homozygous mutation is an identical mutation of both the paternal and maternal alleles.

- Compound heterozygous mutations or a genetic compound comprises two different mutations in the paternal and maternal alleles.

- A wildtype or homozygous non-mutated organism is one in which neither allele is mutated. (Just not a mutation)

By Impact on Protein Sequence

- A frameshift mutation is a mutation caused by insertion or deletion of a number of nucleotides that is not evenly divisible by three from a DNA sequence. Due to the triplet nature of gene expression by codons, the insertion or deletion can disrupt the reading frame, or the grouping of the codons, resulting in a completely different translation from the original. The earlier in the sequence the deletion or insertion occurs, the more altered the protein produced is.

- A nonsense mutation is a point mutation in a sequence of DNA that results in a premature stop codon, or a nonsense codon in the transcribed mRNA, and possibly a truncated, and often nonfunctional protein product.

- Missense mutations or nonsynonymous mutations are types of point mutations where a single nucleotide is changed to cause substitution of a different amino acid. This in turn can render the resulting protein nonfunctional. Such mutations are responsible for diseases such as Epidermolysis bullosa, sickle-cell disease, and SOD1 mediated ALS.

- A neutral mutation is a mutation that occurs in an amino acid codon which results in the use of a different, but chemically similar, amino acid. The similarity between the two is enough that little or no change is often rendered in the protein. For example, a change from AAA to AGA will encode arginine, a chemically similar molecule to the intended lysine.

- Silent mutations are mutations that do not result in a change to the amino acid sequence of a protein. They may occur in a region that does not code for a protein, or they may occur within a codon in a manner that does not alter the final amino acid sequence. The phrase silent mutation is often used interchangeably with the phrase synonymous mutation; however, synonymous mutations are a subcategory of the former, occurring only within exons. The name silent could be a misnomer. For example, a silent mutation in the exon/intron border may lead to alternative splicing by changing the splice site, thereby leading to a changed protein.

Special classes:

- Conditional mutation is a mutation that has wild-type (or less severe) phenotype under certain "permissive" environmental conditions and a mutant phenotype under certain "restrictive" conditions. For example, a temperature-sensitive mutation can cause cell death at high temperature (restrictive condition), but might have no deleterious consequences at a lower temperature (permissive condition).

Nomenclature

A committee of the Human Genome Variation Society (HGVS) has developed the standard human sequence variant nomenclature, which should be used by researchers and DNA diagnostic centres to generate unambiguous mutation descriptions.

In principle, this nomenclature can also be used to describe mutations in other organisms. The nomenclature specifies the type of mutation and base or amino acid changes.

- Nucleotide substitution (*e.g.* 76A>T) - The number is the position of the nucleotide from the 5' end, the first letter represents the wild type nucleotide, and the second letter represents the nucleotide which replaced the wild type. In the given example, the adenine at the 76th position was replaced by a thymine.

  - If it becomes necessary to differentiate between mutations in genomic DNA, mitochondrial DNA, and RNA, a simple convention is used. For example, if the 100th base of a nucleotide sequence mutated from G to C, then it would be written as g.100G>C if the mutation occurred in genomic DNA, m.100G>C if the mutation occurred in mitochondrial DNA, or r.100g>c if the mutation occurred in RNA. Note that for mutations in RNA, the nucleotide code is written in lower case.

- Amino acid substitution (*e.g.* D111E) - The first letter is the one letter code of the wild type amino acid, the number is the position of the amino acid from the N terminus, and the second letter is the one letter code of the amino acid present in the mutation. Nonsense mutations are represented with an X for the second amino acid (*e.g.* D111X).

- Amino acid deletion (*e.g.* ΔF508) - The Greek letter Δ (delta) indicates a deletion. The letter refers to the amino acid present in the wild type and the number is the position from the N terminus of the amino acid were it to be present as in the wild type.

The nomenclature has to cover all sequence variants, descriptions can become very complex. To prevent mistakes and facilitate correct use of this nomenclature, the journal Human Mutation recommends the use of

Mutalyzer, which can apply the HGVS human nomenclature guidelines to check and, if necessary, correct sequence variant descriptions.

Harmful mutations

Changes in DNA caused by mutation can cause errors in protein sequence, creating partially or completely non-functional proteins. To function correctly, each cell depends on thousands of proteins to function in the right places at the right times. When a mutation alters a protein that plays a critical role in the body, a medical condition can result.

A condition caused by mutations in one or more genes is called a genetic disorder. Some mutations alter a gene's DNA base sequence but do not change the function of the protein made by the gene. Studies of the fly Drosophila melanogaster suggest that if a mutation does change a protein, this will probably be harmful, with about 70 per cent of these mutations having damaging effects, and the remainder being either neutral or weakly beneficial.

However, studies in yeast have shown that only 7% of mutations that are not in genes are harmful. If a mutation is present in a germ cell, it can give rise to offspring that carries the mutation in all of its cells. This is the case in hereditary diseases. On the other hand, a mutation may occur in a somatic cell of an organism. Such mutations will be present in all descendants of this cell within the same organism, and certain mutations can cause the cell to become malignant, and thus cause cancer.

Often, gene mutations that could cause a genetic disorder are repaired by the DNA repair system of the cell. Each cell has a number of pathways through which enzymes recognize and repair mistakes in DNA. Because DNA can be damaged or mutated in many ways, the process of DNA repair is an important way in which the body protects itself from disease.

Beneficial mutations

Although most mutations that change protein sequences are neutral or harmful, some mutations have a positive effect on an organism. In this case, the mutation may enable the mutant organism to withstand particular environmental stresses better than wild-type organisms, or reproduce more quickly. In these cases a mutation will tend to become more common in a population through natural selection. For example, a specific 32 base pair deletion in human CCR5 (CCR5-Δ32) confers HIV resistance to homozygotes and delays AIDS onset in heterozygotes.

The CCR5 mutation is more common in those of European descent. One possible explanation of the etiology of the relatively high frequency of CCR5-Δ32 in the European population is that it conferred resistance to the bubonic plague in mid-14th century Europe. People with this mutation were more likely to survive infection; thus its frequency in the population increased.

This theory could explain why this mutation is not found in southern Africa, where the bubonic plague never reached. A newer theory suggests that the selective pressure on the CCR5 Delta 32 mutation was caused by smallpox instead of the bubonic plague. Another example, is Sickle cell disease which is a blood disorder in which the body produces an abnormal type of the oxygen-carrying substance hemoglobin in the red blood cells.

One-third of all indigenous inhabitants of Sub-Saharan Africa carry the gene, because in areas where malaria is common, there is a survival value in carrying only a single sickle-cell gene (sickle cell trait). Those with only one of the two alleles of the sickle-cell disease are more resistant to malaria, since the infestation of the malaria plasmodium is halted by the sickling of the cells which it infests.

DNA STRUCTURE

Deoxyribonucleic acid or DNA, is a nucleic acid that contains the genetic instructions used in the development and functioning of all known living organisms (with the exception of RNA viruses). The main role of DNA molecules is the long-term storage of information. DNA is often compared to a set of blueprints, like a recipe or a code, since it contains the instructions needed to construct other components of cells, such as proteins and RNA molecules.

The DNA segments that carry this genetic information are called genes, but other DNA sequences have structural purposes, or are involved in regulating the use of this genetic information. DNA consists of two long polymers of simple units called nucleotides, with backbones made of sugars and phosphate groups joined by ester bonds. These two strands run in opposite directions to each other and are therefore anti-parallel. Attached to each sugar is one of four types of molecules called bases.

It is the sequence of these four bases along the backbone that encodes information. This information is read using the genetic code, which specifies the sequence of the amino acids within proteins. The code is read by copying stretches of DNA into the related nucleic acid RNA, in a process called transcription. Within cells, DNA is organized into long structures called chromosomes.

These chromosomes are duplicated before cells divide, in a process called DNA replication. Eukaryotic organisms (animals, plants, fungi, and protists) store most of their DNA inside the cell nucleus and some of their DNA in organelles, such as mitochondria or chloroplasts.In contrast, prokaryotes (bacteria and archaea) store their DNA only in the cytoplasm. Within the chromosomes, chromatin proteins such as histones compact and organize DNA. These compact structures guide the interactions between DNA and other proteins, helping control which parts of the DNA are transcribed.

Properties

DNA is a long polymer made from repeating units called nucleotides.As first discovered by James D. Watson and Francis Crick, the structure of DNA of all species comprises two helical chains each coiled round the same axis, and each with a pitch of 34 Angstroms (3.4 nanometres) and a radius of 10 Angstroms (1.0 nanometres). When measured in a particular solution, the DNA chain measured 22 to 26 Angstroms wide (2.2 to 2.6 nanometres), and one nucleotide unit measured 3.3 A (0.33 nm) long. Although each individual repeating unit is very small, DNA polymers can be very large molecules containing millions of nucleotides. For instance, the largest human chromosome, chromosome number 1, is approximately 220 million base pairs long.In living organisms, DNA does not usually exist as a single molecule, but instead as a pair of molecules that are held tightly together. These two long strands entwine like vines, in the shape of a double helix.

The nucleotide repeats contain both the segment of the backbone of the molecule, which holds the chain together, and a base, which interacts with the other DNA strand in the helix. A base linked to a sugar is called a nucleoside and a base linked to a sugar and one or more phosphate groups is called a nucleotide. If multiple nucleotides are linked together, as in DNA, this polymer is called a polynucleotide. The backbone of the DNA strand is made from alternating phosphate and sugar residues. The sugar in DNA is 2-deoxyribose, which is a pentose (five-carbon) sugar. The sugars are joined together by phosphate groups that form phosphodiester bonds between the third and fifth carbon atoms of adjacent sugar rings.

These asymmetric bonds mean a strand of DNA has a direction. In a double helix the direction of the nucleotides in one strand is opposite to their direction in the other strand: the strands are antiparallel. The asymmetric ends of DNA strands are called the 5? (five prime) and 3? (three prime) ends, with the 5' end having a terminal phosphate group and the 3' end a terminal hydroxyl group. One major difference between DNA and RNA is the sugar, with the 2-deoxyribose in DNA being replaced by the alternative pentose sugar ribose in RNA.The DNA double helix is stabilized by hydrogen bonds between the bases attached to the two strands. The four bases found in DNA are adenine (abbreviated A), cytosine (C), guanine (G) and thymine (T).

These four bases are attached to the sugar/phosphate to form the complete nucleotide, as shown for adenosine monophosphate. These bases are classified into two types; adenine and guanine are fused five- and six-membered heterocyclic compounds called purines, while cytosine and thymine are six-membered rings called pyrimidines. A fifth pyrimidine base, called uracil (U), usually takes the place of thymine in RNA and differs from thymine by lacking a methyl group on its ring. Uracil is not usually found in DNA, occurring only as a breakdown product of cytosine. In addition to RNA and DNA, a large number of artificial nucleic acid analogues have also been created to study the proprieties of nucleic acids, or for use in biotechnology.

Grooves

Twin helical strands form the DNA backbone. Another double helix may be found by tracing the spaces, or grooves, between the strands. These voids are adjacent to the base pairs and may provide a binding site. As the strands are not directly opposite each other, the grooves are unequally sized. One groove, the major groove, is 22 Å wide and the other, the minor groove, is 12 Å wide. The narrowness of the minor groove means that the edges of the bases are more accessible in the major groove. As a result, proteins like transcription factors that can bind to specific sequences in double-stranded DNA usually make contacts to the sides of the bases exposed in the major groove.This situation varies in unusual conformations of DNA within the cell but the major and minor grooves are always named to reflect the differences in size that would be seen if the DNA is twisted back into the ordinary B form.

Base Pairing

Each type of base on one strand forms a bond with just one type of base on the other strand. This is called complementary base pairing. Here, purines form hydrogen bonds to pyrimidines, with A bonding only to T, and C bonding only to G. This arrangement of two nucleotides binding together across the double helix is called a base pair. As hydrogen bonds are not covalent, they can be broken and rejoined relatively easily. The two strands of DNA in a double helix can therefore be pulled apart like a zipper, either by a mechanical force or high temperature.As a result of this complementarity, all the information in the double-stranded sequence of a DNA helix is duplicated on each strand, which is vital in DNA replication. Indeed, this reversible and specific interaction between complementary base pairs is critical for all the functions of DNA in living organisms.

The two types of base pairs form different numbers of hydrogen bonds, AT forming two hydrogen bonds, and GC forming three hydrogen bonds. DNA with high GC-content is more stable than DNA with low GC-content, but contrary to popular belief, this is not due to the extra hydrogen bond of a GC base pair but rather the contribution of stacking interactions (hydrogen bonding merely provides specificity of the pairing, not stability). As a result, it is both the percentage of GC base pairs and the overall length of a DNA double helix that determine the strength of the association between the two strands of DNA. Long DNA helices with a high GC content have stronger-interacting strands, while short helices with high AT content have weaker-interacting strands. In biology, parts of the DNA double helix that need to separate easily, such as the TATAAT Pribnow box in some promoters, tend to have a high AT content, making the strands easier to pull apart.

In the laboratory, the strength of this interaction can be measured by finding the temperature required to break the hydrogen bonds, their melting temperature (also called Tm value). When all the base pairs in a DNA double helix melt, the strands separate and exist in solution as two entirely independent molecules. These single-stranded DNA molecules (ssDNA) have no single common shape, but some conformations are more stable than others.

Sense and Antisense

A DNA sequence is called "sense" if its sequence is the same as that of a messenger RNA copy that is translated into protein. The sequence on the opposite strand is called the "antisense" sequence. Both sense and antisense sequences can exist on different parts of the same strand of DNA (*i.e.* both strands contain both sense and antisense sequences). In both prokaryotes and eukaryotes, antisense RNA sequences are produced, but the functions of these RNAs are not entirely clear. One proposal is that antisense RNAs are involved in regulating gene expression through RNA-RNA base pairing.A few DNA sequences in prokaryotes and eukaryotes, and more in plasmids and viruses, blur the distinction between sense and antisense strands by having overlapping genes. In these cases, some DNA sequences do double duty, encoding one protein when read along one strand, and a second protein when read in the opposite direction along the other strand. In bacteria, this overlap may be involved in the regulation of gene transcription, while in viruses, overlapping genes increase the amount of information that can be encoded within the small viral genome.

Supercoiling

DNA can be twisted like a rope in a process called DNA supercoiling. With DNA in its "relaxed" state, a strand usually circles the axis of the double helix once every 10.4 base pairs, but if the DNA is twisted the strands become more tightly or more loosely wound. If the DNA is twisted in the direction of the helix, this is positive supercoiling, and the bases are held more tightly together. If they are twisted in the opposite direction, this is negative supercoiling, and the bases come apart more easily. In nature, most DNA has slight negative supercoiling that is introduced by enzymes called topoisomerases. These enzymes are also needed to relieve the twisting stresses introduced into DNA strands during processes such as transcription and DNA replication.

Alternate DNA Structures

DNA exists in many possible conformations that include A-DNA, B-DNA, and Z-DNA forms, although, only B-DNA and Z-DNA have been directly observed in functional organisms. The conformation that DNA adopts depends on the hydration level, DNA sequence, the amount and direction of supercoiling, chemical modifications of the bases, the type and concentration of metal ions, as well as the presence of polyamines in solution. The first published reports of A-DNA X-ray diffraction patterns—and also B-DNA used analyses based on Patterson transforms that provided only a limited amount of structural information for oriented fibres of DNA. An alternate analysis was then proposed by Wilkins *et al.*, in 1953, for the in vivo B-DNA X-ray diffraction/scattering patterns of highly hydrated DNA fibres in terms of squares of Bessel functions.

In the same journal, James D. Watson and Francis Crick presented their molecular modeling analysis of the DNA X-ray diffraction patterns to suggest that the structure was a double-helix. Although the 'B-DNA form' is most common under the conditions found in cells, it is not a well-defined conformation but a family of related DNA conformations that occur at the high hydration levels present in living cells.

Their corresponding X-ray diffraction and scattering patterns are characteristic of molecular paracrystals with a significant degree of disorder. Compared to B-DNA, the A-DNA form is a wider right-handed spiral, with a shallow, wide minor groove and a narrower, deeper major groove. The A form occurs under non-physiological conditions in partially dehydrated samples of DNA, while in the cell it may be produced in hybrid pairings of DNA and RNA strands, as well as in enzyme-DNA complexes. Segments of DNA where the bases have been chemically modified by methylation may undergo a larger change in conformation and adopt the Z form. Here, the strands turn about the helical axis in a left-handed spiral, the opposite of the more common B form. These unusual structures can be recognized by specific Z-DNA binding proteins and may be involved in the regulation of transcription.

ALTERNATE DNA CHEMISTRY

For a number of years exobiologists have proposed the existence of a shadow biosphere, a postulated microbial biosphere of Earth that uses radically different biochemical and molecular processes than currently known life. One of the proposals was the existence of lifeforms that use arsenic instead of phosphorus in DNA. A December 2010 NASA press conference revealed that the bacterium GFAJ-1, which has evolved in an arsenic-rich environment, is the first terrestrial lifeform found which may have this ability. The bacterium was found in Mono Lake, east of Yosemite National Park. GFAJ-1 is a rod-shaped extremophile bacterium in the family Halomonadaceae that, when starved of phosphorus, may be capable of incorporating the usually poisonous element arsenic in its DNA. This discovery lends weight to the long-standing idea that extraterrestrial life could have a different chemical makeup from life on Earth. The research was carried out by a team led by Felisa Wolfe-Simon, a geomicrobiologist and geobiochemist, a Postdoctoral Fellow of the NASA Astrobiology Institute with Arizona State University.

Quadruplex Structures

At the ends of the linear chromosomes are specialized regions of DNA called telomeres. The main function of these regions is to allow the cell to replicate chromosome ends using the enzyme telomerase, as the enzymes that normally replicate DNA cannot copy the extreme 32 ends of chromosomes. These specialized chromosome caps also help protect the DNA ends, and stop the DNA repair systems in the cell from treating them as damage to be corrected.

In human cells, telomeres are usually lengths of single-stranded DNA containing several thousand repeats of a simple TTAGGG sequence. These guanine-rich sequences may stabilize chromosome ends by forming structures of stacked sets of four-base units, rather than the usual base pairs found in other DNA molecules. Here, four guanine bases form a flat plate and these flat four-base units then stack on top of each other, to form a stable G-quadruplex structure. These structures are stabilized by hydrogen bonding between the edges of the bases and chelation of a metal ion in the centre of each four-base unit.

Other structures can also be formed, with the central set of four bases coming from either a single strand folded around the bases, or several different parallel strands, each contributing one base to the central structure. In addition to these stacked structures, telomeres also form large loop structures called telomere loops, or T-loops. Here, the single-stranded DNA curls around in a long circle stabilized by telomere-binding proteins. At the very end of the T-loop, the single-stranded telomere DNA is held onto a region of double-stranded DNA by the telomere strand disrupting the double-helical DNA and base pairing to one of the two strands. This triple-stranded structure is called a displacement loop or D-loop.

Branched DNA

In DNA fraying occurs when non-complementary regions exist at the end of an otherwise complementary double-strand of DNA. However, branched DNA can occur if a third strand of DNA is introduced and contains adjoining regions able to hybridize with the frayed regions of the pre-existing double-strand. Although the simplest example of branched DNA involves only three strands of DNA, complexes involving additional strands and multiple branches are also possible. Branched DNA can be used in nanotechnology to construct geometric shapes.

CHEMICAL MODIFICATIONS

Base Modifications

The expression of genes is influenced by how the DNA is packaged in chromosomes, in a structure called chromatin. Base modifications can be involved in packaging, with regions that have low or no gene expression usually containing high levels of methylation of cytosine bases. For example, cytosine methylation, produces 5-methylcytosine, which is important for X-chromosome inactivation.

The average level of methylation varies between organisms—the worm Caenorhabditis elegans lacks cytosine methylation, while vertebrates have higher levels, with up to 1% of their DNA containing 5-methylcytosine. Despite the importance of 5-methylcytosine, it can deaminate to leave a thymine base, so methylated cytosines are particularly prone to mutations. Other base modifications include adenine methylation in bacteria, the presence of 5-hydroxymethyl-cytosine in the brain, and the glycosylation of uracil to produce the "J-base" in kinetoplastids.

Damage

DNA can be damaged by many sorts of mutagens, which change the DNA sequence. Mutagens include oxidizing agents, alkylating agents and also high-energy electromagnetic radiation such as ultraviolet light and X-rays. The type of DNA damage produced depends on the type of mutagen. For example, UV light can damage DNA by producing thymine dimers, which are cross-links between pyrimidine bases.

On the other hand, oxidants such as free radicals or hydrogen peroxide produce multiple forms of damage, including base modifications, particularly of guanosine, and double-strand breaks. A typical human cell contains about 150,000 bases that have suffered oxidative damage. Of these oxidative lesions, the most dangerous are double-strand breaks, as these are difficult to repair and can produce point mutations, insertions and deletions from the DNA sequence, as well as chromosomal translocations. Many mutagens fit into the space between two adjacent base pairs, this is called intercalation. Most intercalators are aromatic and planar molecules; examples include ethidium bromide, daunomycin, and doxorubicin. In order for an intercalator to fit between base pairs, the bases must separate, distorting the DNA strands by unwinding of the double helix.

This inhibits both transcription and DNA replication, causing toxicity and mutations. As a result, DNA intercalators are often carcinogens, and benzo[a]pyrene diol epoxide, acridines, aflatoxin and ethidium bromide are well-known examples. Nevertheless, due to their ability to inhibit DNA transcription and replication, other similar toxins are also used in chemotherapy to inhibit rapidly growing cancer cells.

Biological functions

DNA usually occurs as linear chromosomes in eukaryotes, and circular chromosomes in prokaryotes. The set of chromosomes in a cell makes up its genome; the human genome has approximately 3 billion base pairs of DNA arranged into 46 chromosomes. The information carried by DNA is held in the sequence of pieces of DNA called genes. Transmission of genetic information in genes is achieved via complementary base pairing. For example, in transcriptior, when a cell uses the information in a gene, the DNA sequence is copied into a complementary RNA sequence through the attraction between the DNA and the correct RNA nucleotides. Usually, this RNA copy is then used to make a matching protein sequence in a process called translation, which depends on the same interaction between RNA nucleotides. In alternative fashion, a cell may simply copy its genetic information in a process called DNA replication.

Genes and Genomes

Genomic DNA is tightly and orderly packed in the process called DNA condensation to fit the small available volumes of the cell. In eukaryotes, DNA is located in the cell nucleus, as well as small amounts in mitochondria and chloroplasts.

In prokaryotes, the DNA is held within an irregularly shaped body in the cytoplasm called the nucleoid. The genetic information in a genome is held within genes, and the complete set of this information in an organism is called its genotype. A gene is a unit of heredity and is a region of DNA that influences a particular characteristic in an organism. Genes contain an open reading frame that can be transcribed, as well as regulatory sequences such as promoters and enhancers, which control the transcription of the open reading frame.In many species, only a small fraction of the total sequence of the genome encodes protein.

For example, only about 1.5% of the human genome consists of protein-coding exons, with over 50% of human DNA consisting of non-coding repetitive sequences.The reasons for the presence of so much non-coding DNA in eukaryotic genomes and the extraordinary differences in genome size, or C-value, among species represent a long-standing puzzle known as the "C-value enigma". However, DNA sequences that do not code protein may still encode functional non-coding RNA molecules, which are involved in the regulation of gene expression.Some non-coding DNA sequences play structural roles in chromosomes. Telomeres and centromeres typically contain few genes, but are important for the function and stability of chromosomes.

An abundant form of non-coding DNA in humans are pseudogenes, which are copies of genes that have been disabled by mutation.These sequences are usually just molecular fossils, although they can occasionally serve as raw genetic material for the creation of new genes through the process of gene duplication and divergence.

Transcription and Translation

A gene is a sequence of DNA that contains genetic information and can influence the phenotype of an organism. Within a gene, the sequence of bases along a DNA strand defines a messenger RNA sequence, which then defines one or more protein sequences. The relationship between the nucleotide sequences of genes and the amino-acid sequences of proteins is determined by the rules of translation, known collectively as the genetic code. The genetic code consists of three-letter 'words' called codons formed from a sequence of three nucleotides (*e.g.* ACT, CAG, TTT).In transcription, the codons of a gene are copied into messenger RNA by RNA polymerase. This RNA copy is then decoded by a ribosome that reads the RNA sequence by base-pairing the messenger RNA to transfer RNA, which carries amino acids. Since there are 4 bases in 3-letter combinations, there are 64 possible codons (4^3 combinations). These encode the twenty standard amino acids, giving most amino acids more than one possible codon. There are also three 'stop' or 'nonsense' codons signifying the end of the coding region; these are the TAA, TGA and TAG codons.

Replication

Cell division is essential for an organism to grow, but, when a cell divides, it must replicate the DNA in its genome so that the two daughter cells have the same genetic information as their parent. The double-stranded structure of DNA provides a simple mechanism for DNA replication. Here, the two strands are separated and then each strand's complementary DNA sequence is recreated by an enzyme called DNA polymerase. This enzyme makes the complementary strand by finding the correct base through complementary base pairing, and bonding it onto the original strand. As DNA polymerases can only extend a DNA strand in a 5′ to 3′ direction, different mechanisms are used to copy the antiparallel strands of the double helix.In this way, the base on the old strand dictates which base appears on the new strand, and the cell ends up with a perfect copy of its DNA.

INTERACTIONS WITH PROTEINS

All the functions of DNA depend on interactions with proteins. These protein interactions can be non-specific, or the protein can bind specifically to a single DNA sequence. Enzymes can also bind to DNA and of these, the polymerases that copy the DNA base sequence in transcription and DNA replication are particularly important.

DNA-Binding Proteins

Structural proteins that bind DNA are well-understood examples of non-specific DNA-protein interactions. Within chromosomes, DNA is held in complexes with structural proteins. These proteins organize the DNA into a compact structure called chromatin.

In eukaryotes this structure involves DNA binding to a complex of small basic proteins called histones, while in prokaryotes multiple types of proteins are involved. The histones form a disk-shaped complex called a nucleosome, which contains two complete turns of double-stranded DNA wrapped around its surface. These non-specific interactions are formed through basic residues in the histones making ionic bonds to the acidic sugar-phosphate backbone of the DNA, and are therefore largely independent of the base sequence.

Chemical modifications of these basic amino acid residues include methylation, phosphorylation and acetylation. These chemical changes alter the strength of the interaction between the DNA and the histones, making the DNA more or less accessible to transcription factors and changing the rate of transcription. Other non-specific DNA-binding proteins in chromatin include the high-mobility group proteins, which bind to bent or distorted DNA. These proteins are important in bending arrays of nucleosomes and arranging them into the larger structures that make up chromosomes. A distinct group of DNA-binding proteins are the DNA-binding proteins that specifically bind single-stranded DNA. In humans, replication protein A is the best-understood member of this family and is used in processes where the double helix is separated, including DNA replication, recombination and DNA repair.

These binding proteins seem to stabilize single-stranded DNA and protect it from forming stem-loops or being degraded by nucleases. In contrast, other proteins have evolved to bind to particular DNA sequences. The most intensively studied of these are the various transcription factors, which are proteins that regulate transcription. Each transcription factor binds to one particular set of DNA sequences and activates or inhibits the transcription of genes that have these sequences close to their promoters. The transcription factors do this in two ways. Firstly, they can bind the RNA polymerase responsible for transcription, either directly or through other mediator proteins; this locates the polymerase at the promoter and allows it to begin transcription. Alternatively, transcription factors can bind enzymes that modify the histones at the promoter; this will change the accessibility of the DNA template to the polymerase.

As these DNA targets can occur throughout an organism's genome, changes in the activity of one type of transcription factor can affect thousands of genes.Consequently, these proteins are often the targets of the signal transduction processes that control responses to environmental changes or cellular differentiation and development. The specificity of these transcription factors' interactions with DNA come from the proteins making multiple contacts to the edges of the DNA bases, allowing them to "read" the DNA sequence. Most of these base-interactions are made in the major groove, where the bases are most accessible.

DNA-Modifying Enzymes

Nucleases and Ligases

Nucleases are enzymes that cut DNA strands by catalyzing the hydrolysis of the phosphodiester bonds. Nucleases that hydrolyse nucleotides from the ends of DNA strands are called exonucleases, while endonucleases cut within strands. The most frequently used nucleases in molecular biology are the restriction endonucleases, which cut DNA at specific sequences. For instance, the EcoRV enzyme shown to the left recognizes the 6-base sequence 52-GAT|ATC-32 and makes a cut at the vertical line. In nature, these enzymes protect bacteria against phage infection by digesting the phage DNA when it enters the bacterial cell, acting as part of the restriction modification system. In technology, these sequence-specific nucleases are used in molecular cloning and DNA fingerprinting.

Enzymes called DNA ligases can rejoin cut or broken DNA strands. Ligases are particularly important in lagging strand DNA replication, as they join together the short segments of DNA produced at the replication fork into a complete copy of the DNA template. They are also used in DNA repair and genetic recombination.

Topoisomerases and Helicases

Topoisomerases are enzymes with both nuclease and ligase activity. These proteins change the amount of supercoiling in DNA. Some of these enzymes work by cutting the DNA helix and allowing one section to rotate, thereby reducing its level of supercoiling; the enzyme then seals the DNA break. Other types of these enzymes are capable of cutting one DNA helix and then passing a second strand of DNA through this break, before rejoining the helix.

Topoisomerases are required for many processes involving DNA, such as DNA replication and transcription. Helicases are proteins that are a type of molecular motor. They use the chemical energy in nucleoside triphosphates, predominantly ATP, to break hydrogen bonds between bases and unwind the DNA double helix into single strands. These enzymes are essential for most processes where enzymes need to access the DNA bases.

Polymerases

Polymerases are enzymes that synthesize polynucleotide chains from nucleoside triphosphates. The sequence of their products are copies of existing polynucleotide chains - which are called templates. These enzymes function by adding nucleotides onto the 32 hydroxyl group of the previous nucleotide in a DNA strand. As a consequence, all polymerases work in a 52 to 32 direction. ©In the active site of these enzymes, the incoming nucleoside triphosphate base-pairs to the template: this allows polymerases to accurately synthesize the complementary strand of their template. Polymerases are classified just as to the type of template that they use. In DNA replication, a DNA-dependent DNA polymerase makes a copy of a DNA sequence. Accuracy is vital in this process, so many of these polymerases have a proofreading activity. Here, the polymerase recognizes the occasional mistakes in the synthesis reaction by the lack of base pairing between the mismatched nucleotides. If a mismatch is detected, a 32 to 52 exonuclease activity is activated and the incorrect base removed. In most organisms, DNA polymerases function in a large complex called the replisome that contains multiple accessory subunits, such as the DNA clamp or helicases. RNA-dependent DNA polymerases are a specialized class of polymerases that copy the sequence of an RNA strand into DNA.

They include reverse transcriptase, which is a viral enzyme involved in the infection of cells by retroviruses, and telomerase, which is required for the replication of telomeres. Telomerase is an unusual polymerase because it contains its own RNA template as part of its structure. Transcription is carried out by a DNA-dependent RNA polymerase that copies the sequence of a DNA strand into RNA. To begin transcribing a gene, the RNA polymerase binds to a sequence of DNA called a promoter and separates the DNA strands.

It then copies the gene sequence into a messenger RNA transcript until it reaches a region of DNA called the terminator, where it halts and detaches from the DNA. As with human DNA-dependent DNA polymerases, RNA polymerase II, the enzyme that transcribes most of the genes in the human genome, operates as part of a large protein complex with multiple regulatory and accessory subunits.

Bibliography

Bushnell, R.B. . : *Dry Cow Feeding and Management*, A Western Regional Extension Publication, 1979.

Clark, Stephen: *The Moral Status of Animals*. Oxford: Oxford University Press, 1977.

Clymer, R. : *Nature's Healing Agents*, PA, U.S.A: Dorrance Co., 1963.

Daniel L.: *Basic Genetics*, Jones and Bartlett Publishers, Boston, 1991.

Daniel, J.C. Jr. : *Methods in Mammalian Reproduction*, Orlando, FL, Academic Press, 1978.

Daphne C. Elliott: *Biochemistry and Molecular Biology*, Oxford University Press, Delhi, 2005.

Degen, A. A. : *Ecophysiology of Small Desert Mammals*, Springer, New York, 1997.

DeGrazia, David: *Animals Rights: A Very Short Introduction*. Oxford: Oxford University Press, 2002.

Devyani Khemka: *Animal Physiology*, Dominant, Delhi, 2003.

Edward A.: *Papers on Bacterial Genetics*, Boston, Brown and Company, 1960.

Fiore, M. C.; Bailey, W.C.; Cohen, S. J.: *Treating Tobacco Use and Dependence: A Quick Reference Guide for Clinicians*. Rockville, MD: U.S. Department of Health and Human Services, 2010.

Fisher, R. A., 1930, *The Genetical Theory of Natural Selection*, Oxford, Claredon Press.

Frederick B.: *Genetics for Dog Breeders*, Freeman & Company, 1979.

Fridell, R.: *Decoding Life: Unraveling the Mysteries of the Genome*, Minneapolis, MN: Lerner Publications, 2007.

Friedberg, E.C.: *DNA Repair*, New York, WH Freeman and Company, 1985.

Fumento, Michael: *Bioevolution: How Biotechnology is Changing Our World*, San Francisco, Encounter Books, 2003.

Glover, D. M., and Hames, B. D.: *Genes and Embryos*: New York, Oxford University Press, 1989.

Glut, D.F.: *The Frankenstein Legend: A Tribute to Mary Shelley and Boris Karloff*. Metachen, New Jersey: The Scarecrow Press, 1973.

Goodman, D.C.: *From Farming to Biotechnology: A Theory of Agro-industrial Development*, Oxford, Blackwell, 1987.

Gordon, G. A. : *Animals Physiology*, Harper and Row, New York, 1989.

Greene, H. W.: *Mode of Reproduction in Lizards and Snakes of the Gomez Farias Region*, Tamaulipas, Mexico. Copeia, 1970.

Griffin, D.R.: *Animal Minds*, University of Chicago Press. Chicago, 1992.

Grzimek, B.: *Grzimek's Animal Life Encyclopedia*, McGraw Hill, New York, 1989.

Gupta, R.K.: *Freshwater Ornamental Fishes*, Manglam Pub, Delhi, 2010.

Hacker, J.B. : *Nutritional Limits to Animal Production from Pasture,* Farnham Royal: CAB, 1981.

Harrison, R. J.: *Functional Anatomy of Marine Animals,* New York: Academic Press, 1974.

Horn, Toby M.: *Working with DNA and Bacteria in Precollege Science Classrooms,* Reston, National Association of Biology Teachers, 1993.

Hutt, Frederick B.: *Genetics for Dog Breeders,* Freeman & Company, 1979.

John E.: *The Animal Radiations,* The University of Chicago Press, 1981.

Joysey, K. A. : *Development, Function and Evolution of Animal Teeth,* Academic Pr., New York, 1978.

Kurzweil, Ray: *The Age of Spiritual Machines,* New York, Penguin Books, 1999.

Lewis, Ricki: *Human Genetics: Concepts and Applications,* Dubuque, IA: McGraw-Hill Higher Education, 2001.

Lustig, A., Richards, R. J. & Ruse, M. : *Darwinian heresies.* Cambridge, UK: Cambridge University Press, 2004.

Miller, Henry I. : *The Frankenfood Myth: How Protest and Politics Threaten the Biotech Revolution,* New York, Praeger, 2004.

Mindell, E. : *Mindell's Vitamin Bible,* New York, U.S.A: Warner Books, 1980.

Montgomery, G. G.: *The Early Placental Mammal Radiation Using Bayesian Phylogenetics,* Science, December 2001.

Moravec, Hans: *Mind Children: The Future of Robot and Human Intelligence,* Cambridge, Harvard University Press, 1988.

Morholt, E. : *Sourcebook for the Biological Sciences,* San Diego, Harcourt Brace JOvanovich, 1986.

Murray, David: *Seeds of Concern: The Genetic Manipulation of Plants,* Sydney, University of New South Wales, 2003.

Muybridge, E. : *Muybridge's Complete Human and Animal Locomotion,* Dover Publ., New York, 1979.

Old, R.W. : *Principles of Gene Manipulation,* London, Blackwell Scientific Publications, 1989.

Postman, Neil: *Technopoly: The Surrender of Culture to Technology,* New York, Vintage Books, 1992.

Primrose, S.B.: *Principles of Gene Manipulation,* London, Blackwell Scientific Publications, 1989.

Retzer, W.J.: *Biotechnology Workbook,* Englewood Cliffs, Prentice Hall, 1991.

Sayler, G.S., Fox, R., and Blackburn, J.W.: *Environmental Biotechnology for Waste Treatment,* Plenum Press, New York, 1991.

Slater, R.J.: *Experiments in Molecular Biology,* Clifton, Humana Press, 1986.

Switzer, R.L.: *Experimental Biochemistry,* New York, W.H. Freeman and Company, 1977.

Walden, Richard: *Genetic Transformation in Plants,* England, Open University Press, 1988.

Winston, Mark L.: *Travels in the Genetically Modified Zone,* Cambridge, Harvard University, 2004.

Index

❏❏❏